THE BIG BOOK OF
ORGANIC TODDLER FOOD

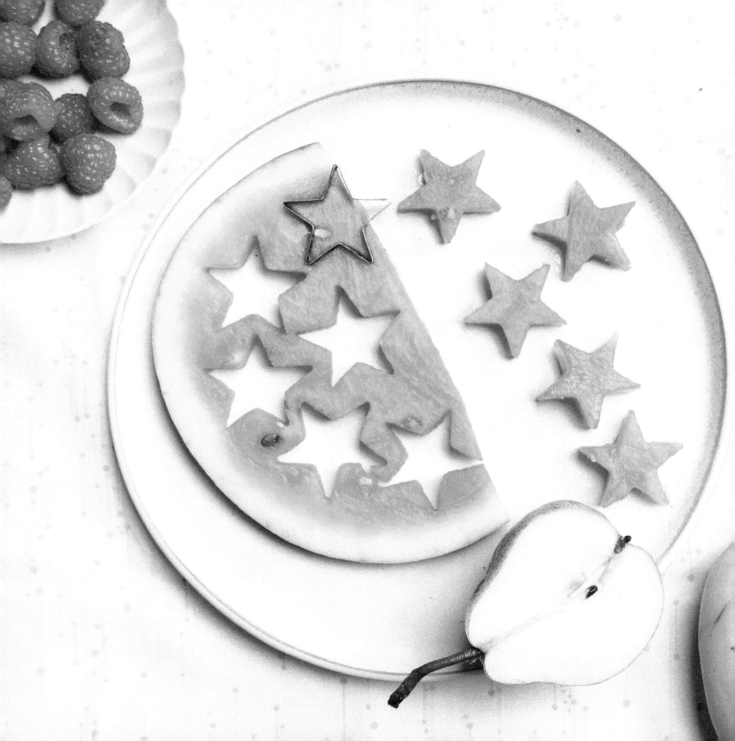

THE BIG BOOK OF
ORGANIC
TODDLER FOOD

A Quick and Easy Cookbook
to Feed the Whole Family

Stephanie Middleberg MS, RD, CDN

ROCKRIDGE
PRESS

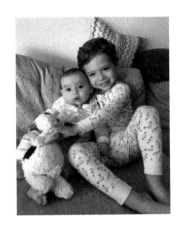

To my toddler son, Julian, the inspiration for this book, and to my baby daughter, Remi, who will soon begin her own food adventures. To my husband, without whom none of this would be possible. And to my parents, who remind me every day what a picky eater I was.

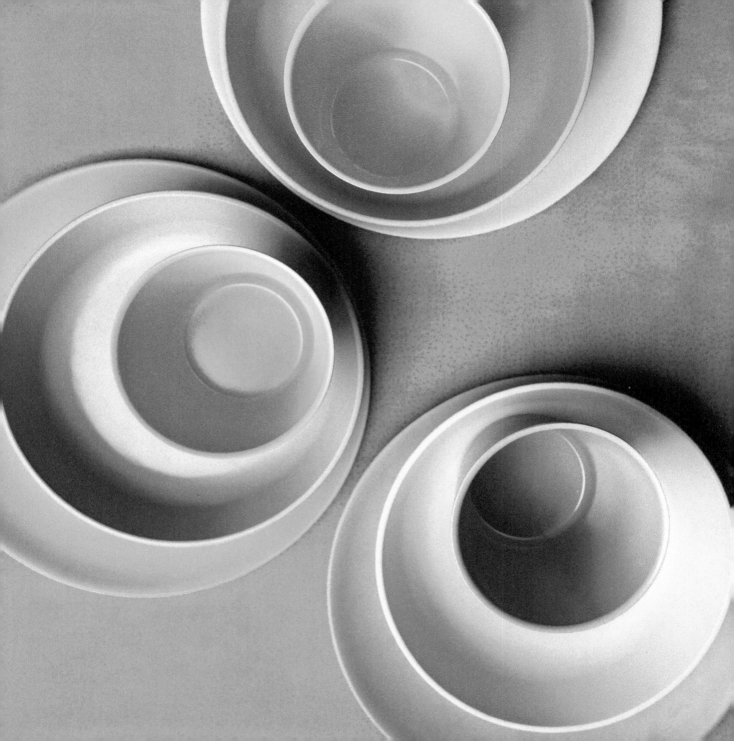

Contents

Introduction xii

Part One: Going Organic and Feeding Your Toddler

1
CHOOSING ORGANIC
3

2
FROM BABYHOOD TO TODDLERHOOD
19

3
FEEDING YOUR TODDLER
31

Part Two: Recipes for Toddler and Family

4
FINGER FOODS 57

5

SMOOTHIES AND BREAKFAST 75

6

SNACKS 99

7

LUNCH 117

8

SIDES 143

9

FAMILY DINNERS 155

10

SWEET TREATS 189

Introduction

My parents were dumbstruck when I told them I was writing a toddler cookbook, even more so when I told them that it includes strategies to prevent and tame picky eating. It makes perfect sense to me: I'm a dietician, I wrote *The Big Book of Organic Baby Food* when my son was a baby, and now he's a finicky toddler who I am responsible for feeding multiple times a day. 1+1+1=3, right? Well, guess what, they couldn't believe I was writing this cookbook because I was a super picky eater as a toddler. So much so that my parents essentially gave up giving me new things to try and my older sister was mortified to go out to restaurants with me in tow.

It's true: For most of my life I didn't care about food. As I got past my picky stage, I just didn't find joy in cooking or eating. I was a terrible first date. Food was fuel, and it wasn't until my then-boyfriend, now husband, lugged pots and pans all the way across Manhattan to my apartment (in his retelling, my kitchen was composed of a stack of paper plates, a pack of gum, and a half-empty can of Diet Coke) that I truly began learning to enjoy cooking and food. I have come a long way since then and my work as a nutritionist is grounded in building and maintaining a healthy relationship with food. This starts with eating real, ideally organic, food, but also includes developing a certain level of comfort in the kitchen, regardless of skill level. As a dietitian, I know there is no healthier option than preparing your own food, and as a former kitchen neophyte I also know how daunting cooking can be. That's why everything in this book is a triple threat of easy, nutritious, and yummy for everyone from toddlers to grown-ups.

But enough about me, let's get back to toddlers. Toddlers are hard! Even the best of them (I was really easy other than eating, I promise, ask my sister!) offer challenges. Feeding a baby, while challenging in its own right, essentially comes down to time management, perseverance, and confidence. That's because babies have no idea what they like and don't like yet. Allergies aside, feeding a baby is mostly about us as parents not projecting our own food issues on them (I'm looking at you, cilantro haters) and ensuring they are getting a variety of healthy flavors and spices. Toddlers, however, are a whole other story. Who better to write this book than a formerly picky eater turned adventurous eater? Mom and Dad: this is the book you wished you had when I was 18 months old.

Everyone asks if my son is an adventurous eater. And the answer is: I wish! He did eat whatever we gave him when writing my first book, *The Big Book of Organic Baby Food*, but my little guy is now a toddler, and you know what that means? He has OPINIONS! Further complicating things is that he developed eczema at four months old and several food allergies by his first birthday, which led to much trepidation on our part to expose him to new foods. During that time, I became increasingly frustrated with the advice we were receiving to best treat his condition. It was always more creams and more prescription medicine that only managed the symptoms of the eczema and allergies. There was little discussion or focus on how to heal or prevent them from getting worse, despite the fact that these are autoimmune issues in which food and nutrition play a central role.

Beyond my own experiences, I am constantly reminded by friends, family, and clients that the struggle to feed these adorable tiny humans is real. Every day I receive questions about what nutrients toddlers need, ideas for fast and healthy recipes for the busy family, and my best tips on reducing pickiness. These experiences are the foundations for this book. We'll cover topics including why organic is important, meal planning, the right amount of food and nutrients for growing bodies, creating a healthy future, and most importantly, making food fun. It's all part of the common thread that toddlers can and should be eating nutritious, homemade food.

This book is a comprehensive resource for you, the parent or soon-to-be parent of a toddler. I'll share over 125 easy, tasty, and healthy recipes that will not only ensure your toddler is eating nutritious delicious food, but that you aren't spending all your waking hours in the kitchen. I hope to inspire you, your family, and most importantly your little one.

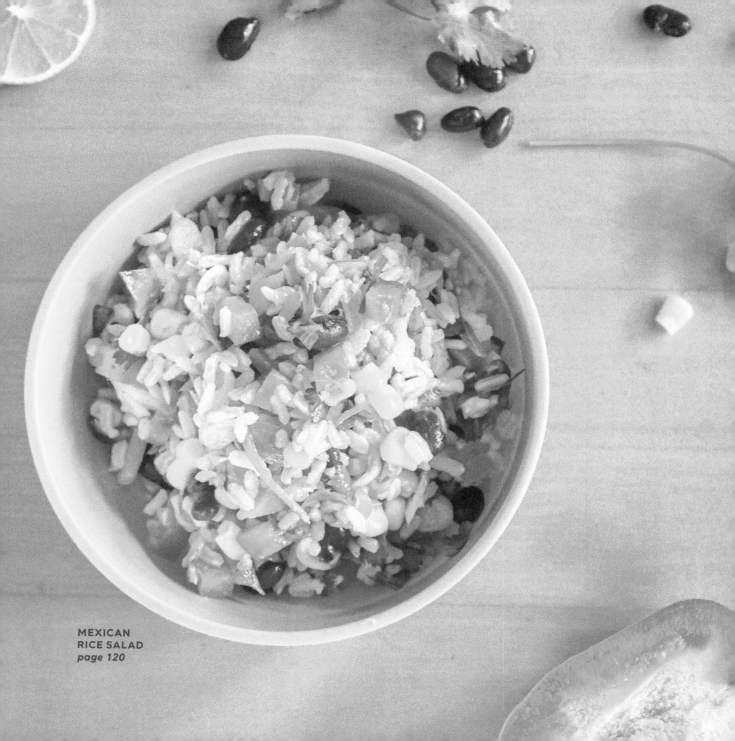

MEXICAN
RICE SALAD
page 120

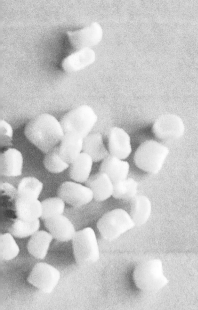

PART 1

GOING ORGANIC AND FEEDING YOUR TODDLER

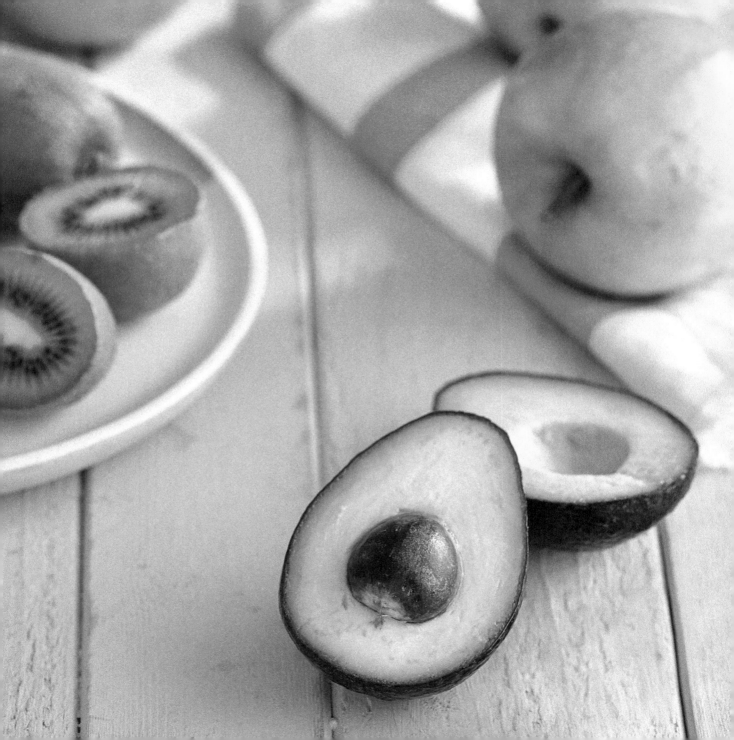

1

CHOOSING ORGANIC

Congratulations on this next step in feeding your child! You've made it to their first year or are nearly there and so much has changed. Just when you've gotten baby food purées down, your wonderful, funny baby grows into an adorable, opinionated toddler. In this chapter, I'll give you the skinny on organic foods and labeling and help you set up your kitchen and pantry for stress-free cooking for your toddler.

The fact that you are already choosing to focus on nutritious, organic, whole foods for your toddler is a major step toward setting them up for a healthy future. Nutrition at this stage continues to be as important as when they were babies. Their digestive systems are still developing and as they transition away from milk toward whole foods, it's important we nurture them from within. It makes a big impact on their guts, immune system, mood (hello tantrums), and those growing brains.

This chapter will set the foundation for this transition, and I'll guide you in what to look for when purchasing food, what certain labels mean, how to stock a healthy pantry, and what tools and equipment you need to make cooking for your family as stress-free as possible. The combination of a more opinionated toddler and introducing new flavors and textures, while also sticking to healthy foods, can be overwhelming to say the least. I'm here to help!

Food is Love

Every parent just wants their kids to be happy and healthy, and there is a certain joy (coupled with a sigh of relief) when they try a new, healthy food and say "more!" Making your own food for your toddler can seem overwhelming and tiring, and it is certainly a labor of love. One day your toddler opens her mouth and says "yum!" and the next day she spits out the same food and refuses

to eat it (I am definitely speaking from experience here). No matter the outcome, keep at it! Things change quickly and the reward is well worth it. Over these pages I'll give you the resources, strategies, and especially the quick and easy recipes to make feeding your family fun!

The Benefits of Home Cooking

I continue to prepare most of my toddler Julian's food because I believe it's the best way to ensure he is eating healthy and wholesome meals, while also introducing new flavors and textures. Don't get me wrong, there are certainly great store-bought and delivery options. Trust me, I use those too, and they're fine to incorporate, but the issue is it becomes almost too easy for them to become the norm, rather than the exception. That's because of a very simple fact: Cooking takes time. Even 30 minutes can feel like an eternity when you're exhausted at the end of the day and you'd rather be snuggled up with your kiddo reading books or playing. But trust me. It. Is. All. Worth. It. Here's why:

NUTRITION

The only way to ensure your child is eating the healthiest food possible is to make it yourself. Full stop. Not only are you picking the best ingredients, but you're deciding how to prepare them. You can sprinkle on some hemp seeds to add a bit more protein or sauté foods using avocado oil to provide a different healthy fat. The possibilities are endless and that's the point. While a bit daunting, this allows you to cater the food to your toddler. If for some reason they have a specific vitamin deficiency, you can fortify the food to combat it (for example, adding a handful of spinach into a soup to boost vitamins C and K). And if your child has food allergies, you can rest easy knowing there is zero potential for cross-contamination. Our son has a nut allergy and it really put our minds at ease knowing that we choose every item of food he eats.

TASTE

Once you start making your own food you really notice the difference in taste, especially the freshness of food that is cooked in season. Taste is especially important to your toddler. While their palate is still evolving, their opinions are really starting to shine through, and the more interesting you can make food, the more likely they're going to want to try it. Plus, their memory has developed, especially for how things taste, so they'll start to ask for foods again and again.

TIME

I've said it before and I'll say it again: Time is the second most important thing in your life right now (sorry honey). And that couldn't be truer with a toddler. Even though cooking for your toddler doesn't seem like it will save time, there are strategies that will make it seamless and stress-free. Most of the recipes in this book can be made in 30 minutes or less and most can be made ahead of time. Plus, there are several slow cooker recipes that can simmer away during the day and be ready to go for dinner. I've got you covered! Once you get the hang of setting a plan, you will find that you will have more time on your hands.

EASE

You do not need to be a pro in the kitchen or need fancy kitchenware to make these recipes. Just like in my first book, the recipes are super easy to follow. Everyone can make these recipes. Plus, my philosophy is to cook one meal for the family so these recipes appeal to kids and adults. We all eat the same meal every night—finicky toddler included.

COST

On a meal-per-meal basis, cooking your own food is more affordable than eating out. It might not seem like that when you're staring down at the cart in the checkout line, but ordering in night after night definitely adds up.

The Benefits of Organic

We all know organic is a good idea, but why? What does "organic" really mean?

The USDA National Organic Program, which enforces organic regulations, defines it as:

Organic food is produced by farmers who emphasize the use of renewable resources and the conservation of soil and water to enhance environmental quality for future generations. Organic meat, poultry, eggs, and dairy products come from animals that are given no antibiotics or growth hormones. Organic food is produced without using most conventional pesticides; fertilizers made with synthetic ingredients or sewage sludge; bioengineering; or ionizing radiation. Before a product can be labeled 'organic,' a government-approved certifier inspects the farm where the food is grown to make sure the farmer is following all the rules necessary to meet USDA organic standards. Companies that handle or process organic food before it gets to your local supermarket or restaurant must be certified, too.

—Consumer Brochure, USDA National Organic Program, 2007.

Choosing an organic start really is the best for you and your family. Here are some of the reasons why.

GROWING BODIES

First, organic foods are grown without the use of hormones, genetically modified organisms (GMOs), and synthetic pesticides. This is incredibly important for little bodies which are more vulnerable to pesticide exposure and other harmful chemicals because their organs and body systems (e.g., digestive system) are still developing.

NUTRIENTS

We now know that organic food contains more nutrients! Organic dairy and meat can contain up to 50 percent more omega-3s and organic produce contains significantly higher levels of antioxidants.

ENVIRONMENT

The world we leave for future generations is another reason to choose organic. By choosing organic, we support growing in conjunction with preserving natural ecosystems and reducing chemical, fertilizer, and pesticide runoff that impacts water supplies, soil, and the larger environment.

Buying Organic

As consumers, we want to eat the "cleanest" foods possible, and we are increasingly interested in knowing where our food is coming from. Demand is outpacing supply and while organic foods used to only be found in select stores, they are now readily available in larger food outlets across the United States. For example, Costco is now the largest seller of organic food. This increase in demand for organic is driving down the cost of organic food.

If cost and resources are a concern, I recommend going organic when you can, and if that isn't possible, check out the Environmental Working Group's Dirty Dozen list (see page 201) and try to avoid those fruits and vegetables on the list. I also recommend you purchase organic for those foods you feed your toddler most often. If your toddler eats an apple every day, try to purchase organic apples. The most important thing is to make sure your toddler has the opportunity to eat an array of foods, even if organic isn't always readily available.

ORGANIC LABELING

Food labels can be completely overwhelming. How many buzzwords can fit into a few square inches? And what does it all mean? This is my profession, and I still often see a new term that makes little sense. It's very easy to go down the rabbit hole and quickly become overwhelmed and nervous about our food choices. The goal here is to be informed and to not let perfect be the enemy of good!

ALL NATURAL: No formal definition exists for this term, but the Food and Drug Administration (FDA) considers it to mean that nothing artificial or synthetic has been added. It is a loose definition, and companies can label virtually anything "natural" so I don't recommend paying much attention to this label.

MADE WITH ORGANIC INGREDIENTS: This means that at least 70 percent of the product must be made with certified organic ingredients.

GMOS AND YOUR HEALTH

By choosing organic foods you reduce your exposure to Genetically Modified Organisms (GMO) that appear in roughly 75 percent of processed foods. The research is young and the jury's still out on the long-term effect of GMOs. What we do know for sure about GMO foods is that they are grown using harmful chemicals, specifically glyphosate and 2,4-D. These have been tied to thyroid, neurological, and reproductive issues, as well as allergies and potentially cancer. Now, I'm not trying to scare you. I'm not saying if you so much as smell a GMO food that you'll get sick—not even close. Sometimes you can't avoid it, and that's okay. I'm trying to equip you with information to make informed decisions. The most frustrating part about GMOs is that we don't always know which foods contain them. Labeling is a work in progress and better regulations and transparency are called for. Because there is no clear labeling at this point, look for items that are certified organic or have the Non-GMO Project Verified label.

THE DIRTY DOZEN

The Dirty Dozen is a list developed by the Environmental Working Group that helps you decide which fruits and veggies are most important to purchase organic. Each year, this advocacy group organization examines data from the FDA and USDA to create their annual Shopper's Guide to Pesticides in Produce, which includes the 12 conventionally grown (nonorganic) fruits and vegetables that contain the highest levels of pesticides—in other words, the Dirty Dozen.

While the Dirty Dozen has the highest levels of pesticide residue, the Clean Fifteen lists the 15 produce items with the lowest levels. I treat these two lists as guides for which produce you should absolutely buy organic and which you can buy conventionally every now and then. Both lists appear in the back of this book (see page 201), but here are the core 12 items on the Dirty Dozen that, most of the time, you'll want to be sure to buy organic: strawberries, spinach, nectarines, apples, grapes, peaches, cherries, pears, tomatoes, celery, potatoes, and sweet bell peppers. In 2018, an additional item, hot peppers, was added to the list, bringing the count to 13.

ORGANIC: This term indicates that at least 95 percent of the ingredients in the product are organic. When it applies to animals it means that they were fed 100 percent organic feed and not given antibiotics or hormones. It also means they were raised in living conditions that accommodate their natural behaviors such as roaming freely, foraging, and not living out their lives in a cage. I recommend pasture-raised organic eggs and grass-fed organic meat whenever possible.

100% ORGANIC/USDA ORGANIC SEAL: A product with this label has been made entirely of organic ingredients.

NON-GMO PROJECT VERIFIED SEAL: This seal verifies that a product doesn't contain genetically modified (GMO) ingredients.

GRASS-FED: This is a label used with beef, lamb, and dairy. Cows naturally eat grass, and their entire digestive system is designed for it. Most conventionally raised cows are fed a mix of corn and other items to increase their fat content (for flavor purposes) and size. Nutritionally, grass-fed animals have higher levels of healthy fats like omega-3s and contain more antioxidants than animals fed a typical grain-based diet. Grass-fed beef is a bit leaner than your traditional cut, but the flavor and nutritional content are immeasurably better.

FREE RANGE: This label is applied to food from animals, but especially poultry. It is a deceiving label because there are no regulations as to how long the animal actually spends outdoors and not in a pen. It could be just a few minutes per day and does not guarantee the animal had access to truly roam freely.

CAGE-FREE: This is another deceiving label that indicates poultry raised without cages. They could be free-roaming and truly cage-free, or they could be living indoors in overcrowded spaces in large factory farms.

PASTURE RAISED: This label is applied to animals who spent some time on the pasture feeding on grass or foraging.

WILD CAUGHT: This applies to seafood and indicates fish caught in the wild, including seas, oceans, and natural bodies of water. You may see some fish labeled as organic but there is no government standard for organic seafood certification. I recommend consuming 2 to 3 servings of fish per week, and choosing those fish low in mercury (especially for pregnant women and children) and high in omega-3s. To find out more about the best fish picks specifically in your state, I recommend checking out the seafood guide by Monterey Bay Aquarium Seafood Watch and the Environmental Working Group.

Eating with the Seasons

Eating seasonally is one of the best things you can do for your family's (and the planet's) health. When purchasing foods in season you'll be eating them when they've been harvested at peak freshness, flavor, and nutritional value. Most of the produce we buy at the supermarket has traveled far and wide to get to us because it has to grow in the right climate. After spending a significant time traveling (sometimes up to five days), produce is placed on the shelves where it may sit for a day or two. And unfortunately, as a result it loses some of its nutritional value and flavor. Let's take vitamin C for instance. In broccoli, vitamin C can degrade almost 50 percent while it makes its way from the farm to your fork. And have you ever had a blueberry from the supermarket in the middle of winter? Yuck!

Unfortunately, mass produce has become seasonless and while that benefits millions of people who would never have access to specific foods (for example, there are no orange groves in Massachusetts), seasons still matter. Eating in season is typically more affordable because food doesn't have to travel as far to get to the grocery store, thus reducing costs. Ever notice how expensive out of season organic asparagus is? I've seen it approach $10 for five stalks. Better to wait until it's back in season or buy it frozen.

The gold standard is to choose organic and local. However, many small family farms can't afford to qualify for organic certification despite following very natural and healthy growing practices. So, the best option for buying in season is to buy from a local farmers' market if possible.

There is something special about bringing your toddler to the farmers' market. It is a great way to expose them to fresh fruits and vegetables. I always have my son pick out a few fruits and a few vegetables to either eat on the spot or bring home. It's up to him and he loves making the decision! He knows the farmers and likes to help us bag everything. We're fortunate to have a farmers' market within walking distance, but for those who don't, not to worry. Include your toddler on your shopping runs. It might take a bit more time, but it's a great winter activity when you're stuck inside.

Here's a list of favorite foods and their seasons. Your list might vary depending on where you live, but this is a good starting point.

All this talk about making sure our toddlers get the cleanest, healthiest ingredients is important, but it's also important to have fun. This is such a joyous time. Don't ever beat yourself up over a meal. Because if worse comes to worst and everything goes wrong, you can always order a pizza! Just don't tell your nutritionist.

SPRING	SUMMER	FALL	WINTER
Asparagus	Corn	Apples	Cabbage
Carrots	Cucumbers	Broccoli	Clementines
Parsnips	Green beans	Brussels sprouts	Cranberries
Spinach	Peaches	Celery	Delicata squash
Strawberries	Tomatoes	Pears	Sweet potatoes
	Watermelon	Pumpkins	
	Zucchini	Winter squash	

A Plentiful Pantry

Now it's time to get into the kitchen! The key to being able to prepare meals quickly is having a stocked pantry. Below is a list of the items that are frequently used in the recipes in this book and some to just have on hand. There are so many choices at the grocery store these days that it can be confusing determining what key words to look out for so I included recommendations. The list below is also what I give to my adult clients so you are not stocking two separate pantries for yourself and your child. While your healthiest bet is organic, if the product is unattainable due to cost or scarcity, don't let that interfere with cooking a delicious meal!

Pantry Items

Almond flour

Baking powder

Baking soda

Cacao nibs

Cacao powder

Chia seeds

Coconut flour

Coconut, unsweetened, shredded

Dates

Flaxseed, ground

Flour, whole-wheat

Hemp hearts/seeds

Honey, raw, organic

Maple syrup, pure

Mayonnaise

Mustard, Dijon

Noodles (soba, buckwheat, whole-wheat)

Nuts (almonds, walnuts, cashews, pistachios)

Oats, rolled

Peanut/almond/walnut/sun butter

Pumpkin seeds

Quinoa

Rice, brown

Tahini

Continued on next page

Cooking Oils/Fats

Butter, grass-fed

Oil, avocado, unrefined

Oil, coconut, unrefined

Oil, olive, extra-virgin

Canned or Boxed Items

Nondairy milk (unsweetened oat milk or almond milk)

Beans and legumes (black, pinto, cannellini,
    chickpeas, lentils)

Coconut milk

Salmon, wild

Tomatoes, crushed

Tuna

Spices and Herbs

Basil, fresh

Cumin, ground

Cinnamon, ground

Garlic, powder and fresh

Ginger, ground and fresh

Mint, fresh

Oregano, dried

Paprika, ground

Rosemary, dried

Sage, dried

Tarragon, dried

Thyme, dried

Vanilla extract

CHOOSING HEALTHIER FLOURS

No doubt you already know that white flour isn't optimal for you or your family. But now that there are so many alternatives available in the grocery store, it can be hard to know what to use and how to use it. Here's a deep dive into some of the options I like best.

If gluten isn't an issue:

WHOLE-WHEAT FLOUR: Whole wheat is higher in fiber than all-purpose flour, and richer in some B vitamins and folate. Whole-wheat flour will give you a heavier result than all-purpose, so start by swapping half in recipes that call for all-purpose. Play around with the whole-wheat/all-purpose ratio to get as much whole wheat in your baked goods as possible while still enjoying the texture. Also try whole-wheat pastry flour and white whole-wheat flour; these are milled from a lighter type of wheat than regular whole-wheat flour, so they have a lighter texture, but you still get the whole-grain benefits.

SPELT FLOUR: High in fiber and iron, this ancient whole grain does contain gluten, but some people find it easier to digest than regular wheat flours. It is lighter than regular whole wheat, and though it has a slightly nutty taste, it's very mild.

OAT FLOUR: This is a good alternative because, in a pinch, you can make your own by grinding up oats in a blender or food processor (use about 1¼ cups oats for 1 cup oat flour). It has a mildly sweet flavor and is very high in fiber and rich in protein and minerals such as magnesium, manganese, phosphorus, and selenium. Oat flour is best for baked goods that are chewy, like cookies. Muffins, breads, and other items that rise can turn out gummy or flat with all oat flour, so combine it with spelt or whole-wheat flour for better results. NOTE: Oats are naturally gluten-free, but unless they're labeled "certified gluten-free," they may contain gluten because of cross-contamination during processing.

Gluten-free flours:

ALMOND FLOUR: Sometimes called "almond meal," it's one of the most common grain-free flours, and it's rich in protein, fiber, and healthy fats. Almond flour and almond meal are simply the nuts, ground up, though sometimes almond flour is ground finer, which will give you smoother, lighter, and less crumbly baked goods. With blanched almond flour, the almond skins were removed before grinding; this will give you a softer, lighter end product (though unblanched is fine if you don't mind a heartier muffin, quick bread, or pancake).

COCONUT FLOUR: Rich in fiber and a good source of protein and healthy fats, this powdery flour is great for grain-free baking because it's mild and slightly sweet, and will give you results similar to regular flour. I recommend seeking out recipes developed using coconut flour instead of trying to swap it in, because coconut flour absorbs a lot of liquid, far more than regular flour or almond flour.

ARROWROOT: I love to keep this light starch around all the time because it's a good thickener (swap it for cornstarch), as well as a binder in baking recipes. Made from a tropical root, arrowroot is rich in potassium and iron, and is best used along with another type of flour (I like to mix it with almond flour and a little bit of coconut flour). Use it on its own in recipes that only call for a little bit of flour, such as crêpes.

CASSAVA FLOUR: Made from the cassava root, this nut-free flour is one of my favorites because it works similarly to all-purpose flour. Because of its flour-like texture and mild flavor, you can usually swap it in 1:1 for all-purpose flour in your favorite recipes. It's lower in calories than almond or coconut flour, but also lower in protein and healthy fats.

ORGANIC CONVENIENCE FOODS

As busy parents, we can't always get a home-cooked meal on the table and need to reach for quick options. We all need backups, as sometimes cooking just isn't in the cards, whether you had to stay late at work or are just exhausted. We've all been there. The good thing is there are perfectly fine store-bought substitutes for a home-cooked meal. Now, as I said earlier, the convenience of these foods can make it very easy for them to quickly become the rule instead of the exception. There are a ton of organic prepared food options on supermarket shelves from brands like Annie's, Earth's Best, Applegate Farms, Dr. Praeger's, Late July, and many more. How can we tell what's actually okay to feed our kids and what isn't? And how often should we be feeding our kids these foods?

The number one rule of thumb is: **READ THE INGREDIENTS LIST.** First of all, less is more; the fewer ingredients, the better. Second, you want to be able to pronounce and understand what the ingredients are. If you are unsure, then my vote is to skip it! While it's certainly okay to have these foods in your rotation, my overall rule of thumb is to keep these items to no more than twice a week to prevent a frozen chicken finger and boxed mac 'n' cheese diet.

As for snacks, whoa! As I sit here typing this my son just walked in the room asking for "orange crackers." This is a huge topic and one that I will cover in more detail in chapter 3 (page 31). As a nutritionist, I'm not a fan of serving "snacky" foods to kids every day. Snacks should be mini extensions of real foods that contain nutrients. An issue I see often is that we tend to over-snack our kids (on not-so-healthy foods) and then they barely touch their nutritious meals. Don't get me wrong, I am also a parent who lives in the real world, and my son does get his organic "orange crackers" from time to time. I certainly don't make a fuss about it, but I also want him to enjoy a snack of pumpkin seeds, hummus and veggies, fruit and organic cheese, and other whole foods to keep it all balanced. And because this is such an important topic, I've dedicated a whole chapter to toddler snack recipes (page 99).

Essential Tools and Equipment

My husband and I have spent countless hours online reading reviews and talking to store owners and friends to find the best kitchen products for our little kitchen here in New York. Below is a list of the items we use the most and what you will need to make these recipes. It's not a lot, but these smart tools maximize efficiency.

PREP

VEGETABLE PEELERS: A sharp peeler speeds the process of peeling your fruits and vegetables and is a time-saving kitchen must-have.

KNIVES: Every kitchen needs one good chopping knife and one good paring knife (and if you're a bread person, a good serrated knife, which also works great to cut tomatoes!)

SKEWERS: Making food fun at this stage definitely helps with getting toddlers involved in the kitchen and sampling foods. Fruit skewers are always a hit! Just cut the pointy tip off before you hand the food to your kiddo.

COOKIE CUTTERS: Because presentation is everything with toddlers, especially picky eaters!

GRATER: We use this to shred certain fruits and vegetables to add to various muffins and meatballs.

COOK

POTS AND PANS: You will need an assortment of pots for boiling, steaming, and other cooking, but you don't need anything fancy for basic cooking. I recommend two saucepans, a smaller one (about 1½ quarts) and a bigger one (about 3½ to 4 quarts). If you plan to make soups, a larger soup pot would be great too. For skillets, one small nonstick, ideally with a PFOA-free surface, is great. You'll also need a larger 10- to 12-inch skillet, preferably a stainless steel one. I also recommend a cast iron pan. It's not as nonstick as a nonstick skillet, but they're usually easy to clean, plus they cook beautifully, they're stove- and oven-safe, and, as an added bonus, the pan imparts some of the iron into your food. Most cast irons come preseasoned nowadays, so you don't even have to take the step of seasoning the pan before using it.

BAKING SHEET: Baking food adds a whole new level to taste. I probably use this in our recipes most nights ranging from vegetables to meats to kale chips and more. You'll want to line your baking sheets with parchment paper, so be sure to buy a few rolls as well.

MUFFIN TIN: I love making muffins. They are such a great make-ahead option and Julian especially loves when I make them mini for him. They make for a perfect on-the-go breakfast or snack. You can use coconut oil to help muffins release from the tin, or purchase silicone mini muffin liners.

Julian loves to fill the muffin tins. It's always his job.

MEAT THERMOMETER: Skip it if your family doesn't eat meat, but I find this to be essential for testing when meat is ready.

BLENDER: You just need one, but get a powerful one that will last. Spending a bit more here is a good idea. I use my blender to make smoothies, soups, purées, dips, blender muffins, and more.

SLOW COOKER WITH A METAL INSERT: Great for bone broth, meatballs, and pulled meats, you can also use the insert on the stove to brown things or as a Dutch oven.

DUTCH OVEN OR A STOCKPOT: Dutch ovens are commonly made of cast iron and can have a porcelain-enamel finish. Brands like Le Creuset or Staub are excellent and built to last. These are perfect for making soups and stews.

SERVE

There are a ton of products on the market catering to kids. I have a bunch of tried-and-true favorites I've listed below, but really anything will do.

PLATES AND BOWLS: I love Avanchy bamboo bowls and plates and spoons. Not only are they bamboo, but they also have incredible suction at the bottom to keep them in place during meal-time to minimize spills. They are also pretty aesthetically pleasing. Dylbug plates are so much fun too. They are personalized plates that your toddler can "dress up" with food. These plates make mealtime fun and can help get your toddler to experiment with new foods in a creative and exciting way.

CUTLERY: I recommend Avanchy spoons and Kiddobloom for stainless steel utensils as well as OXO Tot (great on-the-go) kits. Kiddobloom makes stainless steel utensils in sizes for early toddlers and kids, which are perfect for your little one as they learn how to navigate mealtime with utensils. They come with fun designs, and stainless steel offers an eco-friendly alternative to most of the other plastic options currently available.

LUNCHBOXES: Once it's time to start packing lunches for your toddler, look no further than PlanetBox. It's an eco-friendly, stainless steel bento-box-style lunchbox with various compartments that you can fill up with different foods for your toddler to try. The different compartments are a good reminder to have your child try different foods, as you can get really creative with different combinations! Plus, the quality of these is really unparalleled. I also love the Thinksport Airtight Lunch Container which has stainless steel compartments and a lid that tightly seals for no-leak lunches. They also come with a stainless steel fork and spoon which secure into the lid. I love taking these with us to the park or beach.

TODDLER BIB WITH A CATCH-ALL: Once kids can eat finger foods, I like to transition to a firmer bib with a catch-all so they can munch on the food that inevitably falls. OXO Tot makes some good ones.

CUPS: Munchkin 360 cups are great for transitioning from a sippy cup to a cup. I also love the Thermos FOOGO straw bottles. They are stainless steel insulated straw bottles that keep your beverages nice and cool and fresh for up to 10 hours.

BOOSTER SEAT: As your toddler gets older they like to be part of the dinner table. If your high chair allows, simply take off the tray and push them up to the table. If not, I recommend you transition to a booster seat that straps onto a chair. OXO sells a great one. I find that I still need to strap my son in or he won't sit still long enough to finish a meal.

POUCH PACKETS AND SQUEEZE BOTTLES: These are a great tool for taking your homemade puréed smoothies with you. I don't like to rely on pouches, as they can hinder children's development, but as an on-the-go option from time to time these are a lifesaver. There are a variety of pouches out there, and some even come with spoons like the Kiinde products. I also like Squeasy Snacker and The Original Squeeze Company. They offer a really helpful alternative to single-use squeeze pouches for your toddler. I love that these are reusable and spillproof and they even offer various mouth pieces depending on the age of your toddler. These cute squeeze packs are a portable way to make sure your toddler gets the nutrition he or she needs without having to spoon-feed them.

FREEZE, THAW, AND STORE

RESEALABLE BAGS: Use these to freeze muffins and pancakes, and take along healthy meals and snacks on the go. Stasher Bags are a reusable silicone bag brand, and are ideal for packing up snacks for your little one. Unlike their plastic counterparts, these bags can be used for cooking, baking, microwaving, and freezing. Best part? They are also dishwasher-safe.

ICE POP MOLDS: We love making smoothies into ice pops for nutritional snacks or even breakfasts!

GLASS-LOCK OR PLASTIC CONTAINERS: For finger foods and toddler meals on the go, storage containers are a must. I like Wean Green and OXO Tot.

Okay that was a lot, I know, but we got through it. Trust me, doing the work at the beginning will make things so much easier when it's time to turn the stove on. With the basics covered, we'll now turn our focus to the transition from babies to toddlers. I'll cover going from bottle to sippy cups, reducing milk in your child's diet, signs of finger food readiness, food allergies (a deeply personal topic), beverages, and more!

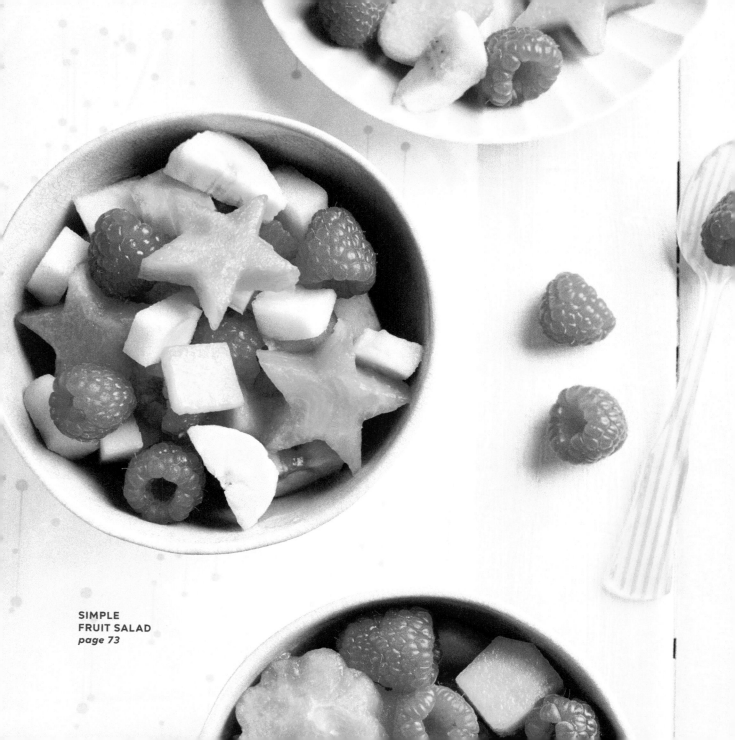

**SIMPLE
FRUIT SALAD**
page 73

2

FROM BABYHOOD TO TODDLERHOOD

Your little baby may now be walking, starting to talk, and reaching for your food! They want to join you at the table and in the conversation. This is such an incredible time, but also daunting. I remember when our son, Julian, decided that he no longer wanted to sit in his high chair, but at the table with us. He wouldn't go in it and we panicked. My husband ran out and bought a booster seat (that Julian was still way too little to really use) and he joined us at the table. It was an incredibly emotional experience. Here was our precious little baby, turning before our eyes into a precious little man! While he could only say a handful of words, he attempted at each point to join the conversation. It was so much fun and we haven't looked back since. So, hold on tight and get ready: Mealtime as you know it is about to change.

Defining Toddlerhood

So what is this mythical "toddlerhood" anyway? Toddlerhood is defined as ages 12 months to 36 months. It's a time of many transitions and a time when your child is beginning to exert their independence. As my son always says, "Julian do it" or his new favorite phrase "by myself!" In this chapter, we will discuss transitions from breast milk or formula to milk, sippy cups, water, and other liquids, as well as food allergies and sensitivities. We also dive into the use of pouches, purées, and finger foods. Some transitions are easier than others, but once you have a guide you will enjoy seeing your little one grow from a baby into a little kid! Much of what comes next is intended as a guide, not hard and fast rules, so do what works for you and your family. For example, my son is well past the purée stage, but we still consistently make them as a complement to his meals, think of it as soup instead of baby food.

Introducing Finger Foods

Finger foods are an important step of your baby's transition to solids. By eight to nine months old, most children should show signs of readiness to eat finger foods, whether or not they have teeth.

SIGNS OF FINGER FOOD READINESS

Babies are ready for finger foods when:

* They are able to sit unassisted
* They no longer gag when offered chunky purées
* They can grab food, first by the fist and eventually between the fingers once the pincer grasp has developed

Contrary to common sense, babies don't actually need teeth to chew. Their gums are really powerful. If you've ever put your finger in a baby's mouth when they are teething, you'll know this to be true! They are perfectly capable of mashing soft foods. In fact, molars don't typically start coming in until 14 to 18 months, and toddlers are eating a large variety of foods by then.

Let them experiment here, as babies love to feed themselves! It's actually very important for their development and promotes good hand-eye coordination. We were very nervous at the start of this phase, but as we began to gain more confidence so did Julian, and it was really adorable to watch him grab and examine his food. A whole new world!

THE SET UP

Have your child seated in a high chair and give him a few pieces of very soft food, about the size of a pea, such as tiny pieces of fruit or very soft-cooked vegetables. Try to avoid putting a full plate of food in front of him, as he'll quickly be overwhelmed and stop experimenting. Set him up for success! Sit with him, SMILE, and be very, very patient.

You may want to start spoon-feeding him, thinking "oh no, he's not getting enough food" or "he's getting frustrated." But let him learn and be there to show support. Trust me, it helps!

As your child progresses past 12 months, you can start to offer a plate with multiple foods that resemble what a fully composed "adult" meal would look like. There are many great options to try at this point and we have a whole chapter dedicated to some fun, easy finger food recipes (page 57). Some basic finger food favorites you don't need a recipe for include:

AVOCADO: Ripe, cut into sticks. I recommend coating them in oat flour for easier pickup.

EGG: I recommend sticking to egg yolks, as they are the most nutritious part. Try hard-boiled and halved or omelet-style and cut into bite-size pieces.

SWEET POTATO: Served without skin, steamed or roasted until very soft.

BROCCOLI: Steamed and broken into large pieces. Florets are easier to gum and great to pair with a yummy dip.

CARROTS: Peeled, cooked, and cut into long thick strips.

A NOTE ON CHOKING HAZARDS

Now for the scary part. Finger foods are a completely new experience for your little one and it is very important to understand that not only are they learning what finger foods are, but actually how to pick up, chew or gnaw, swallow, and digest them. They don't know yet that putting something too big in their mouths is not a good idea. So how do you prevent choking? Here are some easy tips to build your confidence and ensure your little one is never scared of eating:

1. Take an infant and toddler CPR class. Most American Red Cross locations offer them for free. If you can't find an in-person one, YouTube has some great options. However, I highly recommend going to a class in-person, as they will have you practice on a child-sized dummy to build your confidence and knowledge.
2. Try to avoid foods that are roundish like nuts, popcorn, hard candy, and uncut grapes. Your toddler's throat is essentially a round tube so don't give them anything that can block it.
3. Cut food into thin strips. Think thin rectangles, not squares. These will be easier to move down your child's throat.
4. Always, always, always sit with your child when eating, especially in the beginning.

Introducing High-Allergen Foods

Allergies have increased tremendously over the past two decades. In fact, more than one-third of children are affected. And my family is part of this statistic. There is a certain irony for a dietician to have a child with food allergies, especially given I ate really cleanly pre- and postnatally, am in the know, and have little family history of food allergies. The positive is that I've devoted myself to understanding food allergies both to better take care of my child with food allergies and to understand where they come from and how to mitigate and hopefully cure them entirely.

Regardless of whatever side of the allergy fence you are on, diet plays a tremendous role and should be a central focus for dealing with allergies. Many health problems originate in the gut and many childhood conditions, such as eczema, crankiness, sleep issues, and earaches, can be signals that your child may have a food sensitivity.

An allergy is an overreaction by your immune system to a protein that it perceives as a threat.

Your immune system sees these proteins as dangerous invaders and tries to force them out (for example by vomiting, developing mucous, diarrhea, etc.) but it can also appear as inflammation (i.e., redness, pain, or swelling).

The Food Allergen Labeling and Consumer Protection Act identifies the following eight foods as major food allergens:

Milk	Tree nuts (almonds,
Eggs (particularly	walnuts, and pecans)
egg whites)	Peanuts
Fish	Wheat
Crustacean shellfish (crab,	Soybeans
lobster, and shrimp)	

There is growing evidence to suggest that parents should introduce these foods earlier, think around the six-month mark, to combat the potential of developing an allergy. So, then the question is how do you introduce them? How can I give my child something that might hurt them? The answer is simple: slowly, deliberately, and carefully.

Here's what to do. Start very small, with just a taste, not even a full spoonful. Do it near the end of a meal so they are mostly nourished and full. I recommend having plenty of water, a clean washcloth, and depending on your child's history, Children's Benadryl or some other pediatrician-approved antihistamine at the ready (tell your pediatrician in advance that you are going to try the food). Then go for it. If there is no reaction, then the next day, give a bit more, and continue to try the food over the course of a few days, slowly increasing the amount each time. By the third day if they aren't presenting any symptoms they should not have an allergy to that food.

If they do have a reaction, make sure to treat it as quickly as possible, depending on the severity. If there are hives, take a picture for your pediatrician and note where they were, and the severity. Sometimes kids just have sensitive skin and not a full-blown allergy, so it's very important to understand what they can and cannot tolerate. For example, our son had an egg allergy. Working with his allergist we continued to introduce egg in different forms (baked in muffins, etc.) into his diet. Now he has outgrown his egg allergy and loves eating eggs.

THE ROLE OF FAMILY HISTORY

Kids with food allergies don't often get the same allergies as their parents. Oftentimes the parents don't have any significant allergies. But for those parents with significant food allergies, taking steps to minimize allergies in your kids is worthwhile. Pregnant mothers with food allergies should focus on eating a nutritious diet and taking probiotics, bone broth, and vitamin D to ensure a healthy gut. Once the baby is born, consider not introducing solids before four months old.

When Julian first presented with eczema and hives, my husband and I felt like food detectives. After every food we tried, we would observe to see how he acted (since he couldn't communicate). Was he more itchy than normal? Fussy? Could it be he had a bellyache? More gassy? Red in the face? Dealing with kids and allergies is really tough and very hard to pinpoint. But we did keep a journal and slowly we were able to narrow foods down. We don't have many food allergies in our family so these allergies, especially the nut and eggs, were a mystery to us and I didn't know where to turn. There is not a road map for these conditions in kids and there certainly isn't one prototype that works for everyone.

INTOLERANCE, ALLERGY, OR SENSITIVITY?

Food allergies and food sensitivities have overlapping symptoms and a similar root cause—the immune system's overreaction to apparently harmless food. However, there are important differences. The main difference is reaction time. The reaction time of an allergy is fast, within minutes, whereas the reaction time of a food sensitivity is more delayed and can occur hours or days later after the child has consumed the offending food. They both produce fighter proteins with often overlapping symptoms, but only a food allergy can cause an anaphylactic reaction.

Symptoms of Food Sensitivity

These can vary from child to child, but may include the following:

* Skin issues like eczema
* Runny nose and congestion
* Stomach issues (bloating, gas, etc.)
* Sleep issues
* Muscle or joint aches
* Tiredness
* Fogginess

I recommend speaking to your pediatrician or pediatric dietitian early in the process, really as soon as symptoms present themselves. It can be a very frustrating and lonely process to figure out what's going on by yourself, so try to find a practitioner that you see eye-to-eye with. It took me a few rounds to find the right fit. I found it helpful to speak to as many people as possible. But remember, you're the parent and you know your child better than anyone else so be sure to be your own advocate!

Transitioning from Formula or Breast Milk to Cow's Milk

Transitioning from breast milk or formula to cow's milk can be tricky, and I remember needing very clear instructions to wrap my brain around it. It is definitely harder on the parent than the child, as they adjust pretty well. But it is great to have a plan so you're not going into it blindly. See my tips below to help you along the way.

WEANING, WHEN YOU AND BABY ARE READY

Weaning from breastfeeding is a very personal decision, and one that I know many moms struggle with. My advice is to do the best you can. At the end of the day we want to create a low-stress feeding environment. According to the American Academy of Pediatrics, breast is best for at least the first six months. If you can make it to a full year, even better, and if you want to go beyond that, go for it! The ultimate goal is healthy children.

Depending on when you transition, you will need a few strategies, but it's not too tricky. If you made it a whole year breastfeeding that is amazing! There is no need for formula after 12 months so you can certainly begin the transition to cow's milk or other milk. If your child is under a year, you will need to try formula first. When it's time to change over completely, try dropping a feeding a day for a few weeks, being sure to take your time. Then you can start by slowly adding in formula or other milk to the breast milk so your toddler adjusts to the taste, and slowly increase the ratio until you are feeding your child 100 percent of the milk of your choice.

STARTING COW'S MILK OR OTHER MILK

After the age of one, you can start to introduce cow's milk. If there are no dairy allergies, your best bet is to choose organic whole milk. I don't ever recommend low-fat milk for kids of any age. Kids need the essential fatty acids and the fat helps them absorb essential fat-soluble vitamins like A, D, E, and K. If there is reason to think that your toddler isn't handling cow's milk well, then I first recommend goat's milk. We started my son on it, as it is easier to digest (closer in formulation to breast milk), but it also provides all the needed nutrition. If that isn't tolerated well, you could try hemp milk or various nut milks but keep in mind that the commercial brands mainly contain water and not much nutrition at all. The protein, fat, calcium, vitamin D, and other nutrients in nondairy milks are much lower than in cow's or goat's milk. I recommend making your own if you need to use these varieties. Making cashew and hemp milk is actually very easy, and I even show you how to do it (pages 76 and 77)! Of course, when introducing a nut milk you'll have to be very careful to ensure there are no nut allergies.

Start the transition from breast milk or formula to whole milk by slowly adding in whole milk to the breast milk or formula. For example, if your child is consuming 8 ounces at once, start with 6 ounces of breast milk (or formula) and 2 ounces whole milk in the bottle or sippy cup. Try that for a week, then try 4 ounces breast milk (or formula) and 4 ounces whole milk. The next week do 2 ounces breast milk (or formula) and 6 ounces whole milk until finally the last week you have transitioned to a full serving of whole milk.

WEANING OFF THE BOTTLE

The transition from a bottle to a sippy cup should ideally start by around six months so kids have fully transitioned to a sippy cup before their first birthday. It's better for protecting their developing teeth and the earlier you do it, the less attached they become to the bottle as a sleep association. I always suggest doing this in stages, but don't drag it out. Start by switching the first bottle of the day to a sippy cup and go from there with the final transition being the one right before bed. You may want to try a few different brands of sippy cup when starting out because some will be easier or harder to use for each child. A sippy cup of water should start being offered at six months. Drinking from a cup is a skill they need to work on and water is great because it doesn't make a huge mess, children need water at this age, and it can help a lot with constipation, too.

WHICH MILK TO CHOOSE?

Milk is a tricky subject when it comes to our kids' health, and has led to a lot of confusion about options. Should they have it? Should they drink skim milk or full-fat? What about calcium? Are nondairy options real substitutes? Before you decide what to serve, let's break down the pros and cons of all your options so you can make the decision that's right for you! As with many things related to nutrition, there isn't a one-size-fits-all answer.

COW'S MILK: It does a body good, right? Well, it depends on the form. There is a huge difference in nutrition (and taste) between full-fat and skim milk. Full-fat (aka whole milk) is rich in protein and fatty acids, and is an excellent source of vitamins and minerals including calcium, vitamin B_{12}, and riboflavin. Fat is needed to help the body absorb nutrients like vitamins A, D, E, and K and calcium, which are all important for bone health. The full-fat version is also better for blood sugar control. Skim milk is whole milk's watered-down, nutrient-devoid sibling. It doesn't contain healthy fats and fat-soluble vitamins, and often is filled with sugar to make up for the lack of flavor caused by removing the fat.

GOAT'S MILK: Often labeled the "other white milk," it's similar to human breast milk, so it tends to be easier to digest than cow's milk. Goat's milk is also rich in fatty acids, calcium, iron, protein, and potassium. Plus, it's often sourced from small, local farms, which means better quality control and freshness. It's a great option for kids.

NONDAIRY MILKS

There is a huge variety here. Many of these types of milks are lower in protein, calories, and fat than dairy milks so they are not ideal for kids. They are fortified with calcium and vitamin D to compensate for being naturally void of these nutrients. If there is a medical need to avoid dairy then these nondairy alternatives can be part of your child's diet, but you need to ensure your child is getting the added fat, protein, and calories elsewhere in their diet. Always go for unsweetened versions (not the "original" flavor, as these often contain added sugar) and avoid carrageenan. Perhaps most important, read the labels!

HEMP MILK: Made from hemp seeds, hemp milk is naturally higher in protein and rich in omega-3 fatty acids, which are anti-inflammatory and help decrease the risk of heart disease, as well as various cancers and inflammatory conditions.

COCONUT MILK: Made from a blend of coconut fats and fibers (not the liquid found inside coconuts) coconut milk can be found in canned, boxed, and carton varieties. Canned and boxed versions are primarily used in cooking, while the refrigerated cartons are used as a dairy substitute. Coconut milk is rich in lauric acid, a heart healthy saturated fat that has been found to improve good cholesterol (HDL) in the body.

ALMOND MILK: Made by blending almonds and water, almond milk is a good source of vitamin E, magnesium, and potassium. It also has the most versatile flavor, but doesn't contain much protein. While almonds are a good source of fiber and protein, the liquid made from the nuts contains very little amounts of either. Plus, many brands contain carrageenan, a preservative used as a thickening agent and stabilizer. It tends to separate when heated, so it is not the best option to use in cooking.

OAT MILK: A good choice for those allergic to dairy and nuts. It tends to have more protein than the other nondairy milk options.

SOYMILK: The most easily accessible nondairy milk, soymilk is also the most controversial. It provides similar amounts of protein as milk and its consistency is also the most similar to cow's milk. However, it is far from natural. Soy is one of the most commonly genetically modified crops, and soymilk is made with a slew of fillers and contains high levels of estrogen. Plus, many people have undiagnosed soy allergies and have a tough time digesting soy products, specifically soymilk.

RICE MILK: An alternative for people with multiple food allergies including dairy, soy, and nuts. However, it provides little real nutrition.

Water for Life

Up until this point, your child's main fluid intake has been milk of some form. Now, it's time to start adding in water between meals if you haven't done so already. Kids between one and three years old need roughly 4 to 5 cups, or 32 to 40 ounces a day, but their needs vary more by weight than by age. The climate you live in also comes into play with kids in warmer weather locations needing more water. Keep in mind that water can also come from foods that have a high water content like watermelon, cucumber slices, oranges, berries, and cherry tomatoes.

As they get older, healthy children are good about self-regulating their water intake. But in certain situations, like when they are sick or when it's very hot outside, they need more. Kids don't sweat as much as adults, which can put them at risk for heat exhaustion as sweating is a way our bodies cool off. When outside on hot days, aim for 4 ounces (a gulp equals 1 ounce) every 20 minutes or so while outside.

A lot of people ask me about juice. Now my entire nutrition philosophy is rooted in doing your best, not eliminating things entirely, and being realistic. However, juice is the one thing that I just say no to. There is zero reason to give

your child juice, as it's just sugar water. Yes, there are times when they are sick and some orange juice can help. But juice contains just as much sugar per serving as soda and can replace more nourishing food choices, like fresh fruit which provides phytonutrients, fiber, and a variety of other nutrients.

On really hot days or when sick, I recommend making this do-it-yourself electrolyte mix. I actually like to make it into ice pops or put it into ice cube molds for my son. This mix contains all the needed electrolytes without the artificial ingredients. The recipe makes 1 cup.

Electrolyte Drink

6 ounces water

2 ounces of your child's favorite juice (orange juice is a great pick)

⅛ teaspoon salt (I like Morton's Lite salt)

1½ teaspoons sugar (I recommend coconut sugar)

Squeeze of lemon and lime juice

Mix the ingredients together and serve or freeze into pops.

SIPPY CUPS, STRAW CUPS, AND 360 DEGREE CUPS, OH MY!

Sippy cups are a HOT topic. So much thought and money goes into finding the perfect cup for your toddler. And there are so many options! How do you choose? Use this guide to help ease the transition. But remember, every kid is different so it's perfectly normal to need to help them at first. Give them some time to adjust to drinking in a new way.

When to begin?

Sippy cups are meant to transition your baby from a bottle to a real cup. By six months old, you want to have begun to transition your baby away from the bottle. This helps their developing teeth, and the older they get the more attached they get to their bottle. This transition doesn't need to be a "rip the Band-Aid off" strategy. It's okay to take it in stages. Help them with it, and try about two or three different types to find one that works for your child. I don't recommend you let your child walk around with the sippy cup for two reasons: It can be danger-ous if they fall, and too much liquid can fill them up.

Have them drink from their sippy at set times, like right after meals and snacks.

What to look for?

I recommend silicone or aluminum over plastic sippy cups. For first cups, I would choose ones with handles, and most importantly, they need to be leak-proof.

To help with the transition to a cup, I recommend the Munchkin Miracle 360 cup. It comes in a 7-ounce learner with handles and a 10-ounce version without handles, which we used later on. My son loved it and it really prevents messes and spills. They now have a stainless steel option for the 10-ounce cups. If you already have an arsenal of stainless steel cups you like, there are great silicon covers you can put over regular cups. This is also a handy tool to take to restaurants. You can find some of my favorite cups and other feeding recommendations in chapter 1 (see page 3).

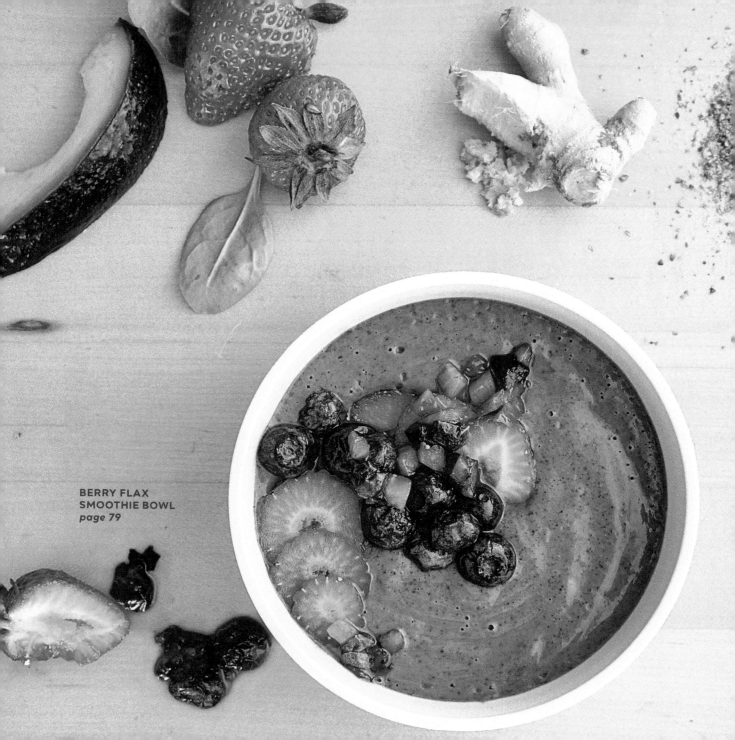

BERRY FLAX
SMOOTHIE BOWL
page 79

3

FEEDING YOUR TODDLER

From nutritional needs to portion sizes, this chapter has everything you need to know to feed your toddler and ensure their proper nutrition. I've also included my tried-and-true strategies for taming pickiness at the dinner table. Your mission, if you choose to accept it, is to cook one meal for the whole family each night.

Toddler Nutritional Needs

What does your little one actually need to eat to grow healthy and strong? I'll break down the nutrients, portions, and information on salt, sugar, and carbs to help you understand what's at stake before you put it on their plate.

VITAMINS, MINERALS, AND OTHER NUTRIENTS

In order to nourish your toddler, it's important to know what vitamins and minerals they need, why, and where to find them in your food.

Iron

Babies have about six months of iron stores in their system so it is very important to introduce iron-rich foods around six months. This is why you see all these rice cereals that are fortified with iron. However, it's important to note that fortified cereals are not great sources of iron, as they are not absorbed efficiently. It's more ideal to offer your child whole iron-rich foods like meats and bone broth instead. For those who are anemic or at risk for being anemic, I recommend separating calcium and iron sources at meals, as calcium inhibits the absorption of iron.

FOOD SOURCES: Iron is found in both animal and plant foods. There are two forms of iron found in food, heme and non-heme. Heme iron comes from animal protein, mainly meat, whereas non-heme iron comes from plant-based foods and isn't absorbed as well. Most absorbable sources of iron come from meat, poultry, and fish. Vegetarian sources include legumes, tofu, and green leafy vegetables. Additionally, vitamin C helps with the absorption of iron so including fruits and veggies in your child's meal is ideal. A good combo includes spaghetti squash with ragu sauce and sautéed spinach or chicken and broccoli. Other sources of iron include organic blackstrap molasses (add a tablespoon to smoothies) and bone broth to add as a base to soups.

Probiotics

Your child's gut health directly impacts how they feel every day and is important for overall health. A healthy intestinal flora is key for efficient digestion function and a strong immune system. Increasing your little one's good gut bacteria not only reduces constipation, but can also improve issues with gas, colic, and acid reflux. It can also improve or reduce the likelihood of some common kid conditions like eczema, food allergies, and asthma.

FOOD SOURCES: You can get probiotics from food sources, primarily fermented foods like fermented veggies (think sauerkraut but also made with other veggies like beets, carrots, etc.), which can be found in the refrigerated section of many grocery stores. Other sources include yogurt, kefir, and miso. You can also start them on a powder supplement as early as a few months. We added ¼ teaspoon of powder supplement to the breast milk we fed Julian.

The level and type of "bad" bacteria your baby is exposed to early on can have an impact on whether they develop one of the three common chronic conditions: allergies, asthma, and eczema.

Consider giving your little one a supplement if:

* Your baby was born via C-section
* You or your baby were given antibiotics or steroids early on
* You had antibiotics during pregnancy, delivery, or while nursing

Vitamin D

Vitamin D is important for everyone as it helps boost bone mass and mineralization, the immune system, and overall mood. It can also help protect against illness such as common colds, respiratory infections, and the flu.

FOOD SOURCES: Vitamin D is found in animal products (especially in liver and egg yolks) but 20 minutes of sun exposure each day is really the best way for the body to produce enough of this vitamin. However, anyone living in areas with little sunlight during the winter months will want to consider taking a supplement. According to the American Academy of Pediatrics, breastfed babies under 12 months need to take a daily 400 IU vitamin D supplement. Vitamin D is already added to baby formula, which is why formula-fed babies don't need the supplement. You get it in a liquid form and it can be added to breast milk or formula or simply placed in their mouth. Children over 12 months old need 600 IU, but some children could need more especially if they live in areas with little sunlight. Cod liver oil is a good source of vitamin D.

Fats

Fat is essential for toddlers' growing bodies. Did you know that breast milk is made of roughly 60 percent fat and cholesterol? Fats help absorb fat-soluble vitamins (like A, D, E, and K) and are essential for brain and nerve development. In addition to ensuring fat-soluble vitamins, antioxidants, and minerals will be absorbed, fat also keeps blood sugar balanced, promotes healthy skin and cells, keeps us more "full," and provides us with antiviral and antimicrobial benefits. Perhaps most importantly when it comes to feeding toddlers, it tastes great, too! You never need to choose a low-fat product for your child. They typically contain more sugar and additives. Plus, your kid needs the fat!

FOOD SOURCES: Include healthy fats like avocado, nut butters, seeds (pumpkin, sunflower, etc.), oils (extra-virgin olive oil, coconut oil, and avocado oil), ghee, and full-fat dairy.

Omega-3 Fatty Acids

This essential fatty acid is important for brain development, and has beneficial effects on numerous neurological disorders such as ADHD, autism, dyslexia, and aggression.

FOOD SOURCES: The best source of omega-3 fatty acids are cold-water fishes like salmon, anchovies, and sardines. The omega-3s in these fish are more readily absorbed by the body than plant-based forms like flaxseed, chia seeds, and walnuts. Since sardines and anchovies aren't necessarily the most appetizing (but hey, try them . . . even in a dressing), I recommend serving these types of fish in addition to others like wild flounder, sole, cod, and halibut at least twice a week. In general, the smaller the fish, the less mercury it contains. Fish also are rich in key nutrients like selenium, zinc, and copper.

Kids should minimize their intake of the higher mercury fish, such as yellowfin and canned albacore tuna, Spanish and king mackerel, Chilean sea bass, marlin, orange roughy, shark, swordfish, and bigeye/ahi tuna.

My favorite resources to help educate you on which seafood to choose are Monterey Bay Aquarium Seafood Watch and Environmental Working Group's Consumer Guide to Seafood.

Zinc

Zinc is helpful for keeping your toddler's immune system strong and their skin resilient. A baby's stores of zinc deplete by around six months.

FOOD SOURCES: The main sources of zinc are found via animal products. Oysters contain more zinc per serving than any other food, but red meat and poultry provide the majority of zinc in the American diet. Other good sources of zinc include beans, nuts, certain types of seafood (such as crab and lobster), eggs, whole grains, tofu, and dairy products. Sprouting grains may increase bioavailability of zinc.

Calcium

Calcium is key for skeletal and bone development.

FOOD SOURCES: Full-fat and fermented dairy products are great sources if there are no signs of reaction to dairy: no skin breakouts, digestive issues, or sinus congestion. Goat milk is another wonderful source of calcium, especially for those who can't tolerate cow's milk. Nondairy sources include beans, dried figs, sweet potatoes, Swiss chard, kale, collards, mustard greens, some brands of tofu, and sesame seeds.

NOURISHING FOODS

These are foods that are incredibly healthy for a variety of reasons.

BONE BROTH: Bone broths are an easy way to enrich your family's diet with minerals and other healing nutrients, as well as improve overall digestion. Bone broth is a nutrient-rich and flavorful mixture made by boiling bones of healthy animals with vegetables, herbs, and spices for an extended period of time (once upon a time we called this stock, and now you know why people serve chicken soup when you're sick—it's not the chicken or the noodles!). It's been popping up everywhere and for good reason. It's delicious and comforting and has become known as a bit of a cure-all, as it builds strong bones, boosts the immune system, improves digestion, and supports joints, hair, skin, and nails. Whenever our son is sick, we make him bone broth (or purchase it ready-made from a local source) and mix in quinoa and shredded chicken.

Broth is an excellent source of calcium, magnesium, and phosphorus, which makes it great for our bones and teeth. It is rich in chondroitin and glucosamine which is good for our joint health and inflammation, and glutamine and other amino acids that are especially healing to the gut and thus help nutrient absorption and your immune system. Proper nutrition is more than what we eat, but how well our bodies absorb what we eat. When purchasing broth, choose products that are made from organic and/or grass-fed sources. Or make your own (see page 160).

COD LIVER OIL: In addition to supplying DHA and EPA, it's incredibly rich in vitamins A and D (which is very tough to get through food). It's a powerhouse for preventing inflammation and chronic disease and is incredible for your child's immune system and brain development.

REAL TALK ABOUT VEGETABLES

Getting kids to eat their veggies is by far the biggest food challenge we face as parents. This is likely one of the reasons you bought this book. So let's get into it!

Patience, persistence, and playfulness are the keys to vegetable consumption. You don't have to offer veggies in one particular way.

Think outside of the box and play around with some fun ideas to make these nutritious foods part of your meals. At the same time, be sure to remain gentle and not become upset or stop offering them when they end up on the floor or still on the plate.

You may want to start by offering cooked vegetables. Yes, kids can tolerate raw veggies (they did for thousands of years) but cooking things will improve the flavor and make them easier to digest. Steaming is still a great method to ensure peak nutritional value, but let's be honest, steamed veggies plain aren't very tasty or exciting. This is a great time to introduce fats when cooking (remember, your child needs fat for brain development). Think grass-fed butter, olive, avocado, and coconut oils, and ghee (clarified butter). Try roasting veggies with oil and seasonings and cut them into fries or chips. Blending veggies into bone broth–based soups is another easy way to introduce new vegetables into your family's diet. We sauté spinach and onions, and blend this together with bone broth for an easy soup Julian loves. Adding chopped and sautéed bell peppers, cabbage, onions, and/or carrots into a morning scramble is another simple way to up your vegetable offerings. Sauté zucchini rounds in butter with a bit of salt and spice powder for a nutritious finger food, or add veggies into classic meat dishes like shredded

SPOTLIGHT ON VEGETARIAN DIETS

When raising a healthy vegetarian, you need to ensure your toddler will be getting all the essential nutrients. The main nutrients to focus on are B_{12}, zinc, iron, vitamin D, and protein. Knowing which vegetarian-friendly foods are good sources of these key nutrients is important, but every child is different so it's important to talk to your pediatrician or a dietitian to get a full assessment and recommendations for your individual child.

IRON:

* Black beans
* Blackstrap molasses
* Broccoli
* Dark leafy greens (kale, Swiss chard, and collard greens)
* Dried apricot
* Lentils
* Oatmeal
* Peas
* Spirulina
* Tofu

ZINC:

* Eggs
* Legumes
* Pumpkin seeds
* Tofu
* Wheat germ

VITAMIN B_{12}:

* Eggs
* Hard cheese
* Milk (if 12 months +)
* Nutritional yeast

PROTEIN:

There are plenty of protein options for vegetarian toddlers. Choose whole foods and skip the fake-meat alternatives that are filled with processed soy and preservatives.

* Cheese
* Edamame
* Hemp seeds/hearts
* Legumes
* Nuts/nut butters
* Quinoa
* Seeds (pumpkin, sunflower)
* Spirulina
* Tofu
* Yogurt

VITAMIN D:

Sunshine is really the best source, so you most likely will want to consider supplementation if getting daily sunshine is an issue.

SUPERFOODS

These are nutrient-rich foods that not only provide your toddler with health benefits but also help prevent chronic diseases and boost their immune system. This book is filled with superfoods with an emphasis on providing your toddler with a mega dose of nutrition. Some of the most common superfoods include leafy greens like kale and spinach, seeds like chia, flaxseed, and pumpkin, and other wide-ranging foods such as avocado, sweet potatoes, pumpkin, salmon, and berries. The recipes in this book are filled with fat-soluble vitamins (A, D, E, and K) to assist with absorption of these superfoods.

carrots and zucchini in meatloaf, mushrooms in beef or turkey burgers, or shredded zucchini and carrot in a beef lasagna. They are still getting the flavor of and exposure to the vegetable, which is the most important part. In terms of introducing raw veggies, my son loves raw carrots dipped in hummus, which are a bit more fun for him to eat. I also serve these at the start of the meal as an appetizer when he is most hungry. Or you can add raw veggies to smoothies.

You can also involve your toddler in food shopping and food prep, which often leads to

taste-testing. See Preventing and Taming Picky Eaters (page 43) for more ideas. Finally, I find it helps to read books about vegetables—the more interesting they seem the more interested your toddler will be in trying them.

Rest assured, it's very normal for your toddler to not love veggies. Rejecting vegetables is a stage and they will start to like them again later on. The important thing is to offer them at every meal so they get used to these nutritious and delicious foods.

My favorite ways to eat veggies include:

1. Kale Chips (page 115)
2. Spinach in smoothies, such as Fruit and Greens Smoothie (page 82)
3. Blending veggies with bone broth for soups or purées, (they're not just for babies!)
4. Veggie Noodles (Zoodles) (page 145)
5. Zucchini or squash in meatballs, such as in Turkey and Veggie Meatballs (page 134)
6. Mini Zucchini Pizzas (page 71)
7. Smashed Cauliflower (see page 148) or Cauliflower Rice (see page 144)
8. Cauliflower Tots (page 62)
9. Veggies and dip (sliced cucumber or red, green, or yellow peppers with Citrus-Tahini Dipping Sauce [page 104], Zucchini Dip [page 111], Lemon-Yogurt Dipping Sauce [page 166], or hummus)

ANATOMY OF A SMOOTHIE

While we are on the subject of vegetables, let's talk about smoothies, as they are a great vehicle for bulking up the fruits and veggies in your child's diet in a fun way. I always encourage a little experimentation in the kitchen. If you generally go by the (recipe) book, smoothies are the perfect departure for winging it with confidence. Every great smoothie starts with a liquid and fresh or frozen produce. It's only improved by the additions of protein and healthy fat (which make an ideal base), and a superfood or two.

FOR A STARTER SMOOTHIE, choose one ingredient each from the liquid and base columns, and one to three ingredients from the fruit column.

FOR A GREEN SUPER SMOOTHIE, choose one ingredient each from the liquid, base, and vegetables columns. Feel free to use a combination of fruits and more than one add-in.

Save that Smoothie

TOO THICK: Add more liquid. Start with ¼ cup and add in ¼-cup increments.

TOO THIN: Add more fruit or yogurt.

TOO BITTER: Sweeten by adding 1 Medjool date or 1 teaspoon of raw honey (for children over 12 months), pure maple syrup, or pure vanilla extract.

TOO WARM: Add a handful of ice.

NOT BLENDING WELL: Blend in batches in this order: liquid, greens, fruit, add-ins.

LIQUID	BASE	FRUIT	VEGETABLES	SUPERFOOD ADD-INS
1 cup	1 to 2 tablespoons	1 to 2 cups	1 to 2 handfuls	1 to 2 tablespoons seeds or ¼ teaspoon herbs and spices
Cow's milk	Nut butters	Banana	Kale	Chia seeds
Nondairy milk (coconut, almond, oat, etc.)	Yogurt or kefir	Berries	Spinach	Flaxseed
Water or coconut water	Avocado	Pear	Chard	Hemp seeds
	Tofu	Mango	Cucumber	Wheat germ
	Collagen powder	Cherries	Zucchini	Mint
		Pineapple	Carrots	Basil
		Your choice!	Cauliflower	Ginger
			Beets	Turmeric

TODDLER PORTIONS

How much should my toddler be eating at a meal is a question I get all the time. Remember, you control what is being served, but let your child lead the way on how much they consume. Just like with adults, I don't recommend ever counting calories with kids. Toddlers are incredibly good at knowing when they have had enough so they really are able to stop when full and ask for more when hungry. They may eat voraciously one day and hardly at all the next day.

Think about their food consumption more on a week-to-week basis than day-to-day. Let them lead. They will get what they need. Most of us adults have lost the innate ability to listen to our body's cues of fullness so it can be baffling at times to see your little one leave two bites of food (or more) on their plate, but when they are done they are done (or maybe they just need a break to play).

Next is a portion guideline for toddlers, but the amounts will vary with each child and from meal to meal. Sometimes my son can have a full six-ounce fillet of salmon and the next day he will eat just half that amount. When guesstimating toddler portions, think of them as one-quarter to one-half the size of an adult portion.

TODDLER PORTION SIZES:

* Vegetables: 2 to 3 tablespoons
* Fruits: ½ fresh fruit
* Grains: 2 to 4 tablespoons
* Animal Proteins: 1 to 3 ounces
* Legumes: 2 tablespoons

PORTIONING TIPS:

* Always offer a smaller amount on their plate at first so as to not overwhelm them, and then you can provide more when they ask.
* Offer three meals per day with one to two snacks.
* Serve protein at every meal and ideally with at least one snack.
* Serve veggies and fruit at two to three meals per day and with at least one snack.
* Serve complex carbohydrate grains one to three times per day.

THE SKINNY ON SUGAR AND SALT

When Julian was a baby I worked hard so that he'd develop a more "savory" palate and stayed away from sugar as much as possible. But as he has gotten older he is of course exposed to it at parties, at preschool, and with his friends, and I have to take a more realistic approach. Refined sugar in the form of desserts isn't in his diet often but it is important for us to enjoy all foods and that means getting ice cream once in a while (I think there is nothing cuter than watching a little kid eat ice cream). But the key is knowing the different forms of sugar, the sources, and how often to offer it, not to eliminate it altogether. Trust me, eliminating sweets altogether will backfire.

So let's back up. Sugar comes in two forms. The first is the naturally occurring sugars found in fruits, vegetables, and dairy products. These are perfectly fine and I don't recommend limiting these forms, as these foods are also loaded with many vitamins, minerals, and fiber. Even dried fruits like raisins and freeze-dried fruits are great to add diversity so long as the dried fruit has no added sugar or sulfites and it's not replacing fresh fruit intake. Also, these can be a choking hazard depending on the age so parents need to be watchful. I love adding freeze-dried fruits to yogurt or on top of a smoothie as "sprinkles."

The second form is added and refined sugars that are not naturally present in food and this is the category to limit. What's the issue with added sugar? First, kids are simply eating more sugar than ever before. It affects both your child's immune system and their digestion. It can also lead to low blood sugar and a case of the "hangries" or mood issues associated with it. Plus, sugar can be highly addicting. It's amazing how after you have it one day you feel like you need it the next.

Added sugars are not only found in dessert foods like cookies, cake, and ice cream and beverages like soda and juice, but also can be hidden in "healthy" foods like yogurt, cereal, granola, granola bars, and oatmeal.

The American Heart Association recommends a maximum of 6 teaspoons (25 grams) of added sugar a day for kids 2 to 18 years of age and 0 grams of added sugar for those under the age of 2.

See how quickly that can add up:

5.3-ounce container sweetened yogurt = 3 teaspoons of added sugar

Granola bar = 2 to 3 teaspoons of added sugar

4 ounces juice = 2½ teaspoons of added sugar

Ketchup: 1 tablespoon serving = 1 teaspoon of added sugar

2 waffles = 1 teaspoon of added sugar

The good news is that manufacturers now have to list added sugars on the nutrition labels so we can more easily differentiate natural from added sugars.

Here are some tips on how to manage sugar consumption:

* Make sure breakfast is packed with protein and fat. We wake up with our blood sugar at its lowest so feeding it with sugar first thing will only cause our blood sugar to crash more, leading to craving more sugar and making us moody.
* When having some sugar, try to include it with a protein and/or fat to slow its absorption. For example, if using maple syrup in oatmeal include a protein or fat like some nuts, seeds, or nut butter.
* Purchase unsweetened foods whenever possible so that you can sweeten them yourself. That way you can control how much

sweetener is added. In items like yogurt, I love thawing frozen berries to make a "jam" as well as putting dried fruit in water and then blending and using as a "jam" rather than purchasing fruit yogurts. Or if using maple syrup or honey, try keeping portions to a teaspoon.

* Use these natural sweeteners instead of processed sugar: dates, pure maple syrup, and raw honey (after age 12 months). I also recommend using coconut sugar in baked recipes. These sweeteners are all healthier than any other forms of refined sugar, as they contain nutrients and don't spike blood sugar the same way as processed forms do.
* Read the ingredients on food labels to determine if sugars are being added. Look for added sugar ingredients like cane sugar, corn sweetener, high-fructose corn syrup, fruit juice concentrate, molasses, and any ingredient ending with an "ose."
* Avoid making desserts rewards or bribes and a daily occasion.
* Mix up sweet and savory dishes—try the Oat and Cranberry Breakfast Cookies (page 86) one day and Broccoli and Cheese Mini Frittata Muffins (page 85) for breakfast the next day.
* Try to avoid making it a big deal when your toddler has a treat. Just enjoy it!

With regard to salt, food for your toddler shouldn't be bland. Kids should be exposed to a variety of flavors. In fact, this helps them become more adventurous eaters later on in life. After the age of 12 months, salt is fine to use but you don't need to have a heavy hand as a small amount goes a long way. When cooking, I recommend using fine sea salt. Try using herbs and spices in your cooking to maximize flavor. I particularly love cinnamon, ginger, cumin, tarragon, garlic, and onion powder, but there are many more to experiment with, too!

SNACKING RIGHT

This is probably my favorite topic to chat about. Maybe it's because I am a snacker myself and love my snacks! Kids love them too. But with so many choices it can be tough to know which ones are healthy. When I work with adults and families, often meals are super nutritious but snacks tell a different story and these "in-between" eating occasions can make a big difference. Snacks are important to help control blood sugar and mood in kids. The key is to look at snacks as extensions of a meal, meaning ensuring you are providing nutritionally dense foods. An ideal snack contains protein, fiber, and fat. Some snack ideas that include all three are below.

AT-HOME SNACKS

* Pumpkin Energy Balls (page 108)
* Banana Sushi Bites (page 110)
* Veggies and hummus
* Fruit and nut butter
* Yogurt parfait
* Ants on a log (celery with nut butter or sun butter and raisins)

* Apple Sandwiches with Cashew Butter (page 92)
* Edamame

ON-THE-GO SNACKS
* Pumpkin seeds
* Fresh fruit and string cheese
* Seaweed snacks and hummus
* Nut butter packets
* Roasted chickpeas
* Plain whole-milk yogurt
* Beef, salmon, or turkey jerky

* Kale Chips (page 115)
* Homemade muffins or granola bars (page 105)

The next question is how often should your toddler be snacking? It's key to set a snack schedule to avoid grazing. Ideally you are giving a snack between breakfast and lunch and another between lunch and dinner. Sometimes kids will have growth spurts where they just have hungrier days so it's perfectly fine to offer more.

DON'T CUT THE CARBS

We've already covered how important fat is for growing bodies (see page 33). Another topic of concern with parents is whether they should give their toddlers carbohydrates. The short answer is yes because growing kids are constantly expending energy, whether during play or a growth spurt, and their bodies need fuel to support and nourish them. But not all carbs are the same!

Simple carbohydrates are your starchy items like white bread, white rice, and white pasta. Basically, anything made with white flour falls in this category. Simple carbs lack fiber and are broken down into sugar, which the body uses for energy very quickly. These foods tend to cause a fast energy spike and a fast crash, making you feel more tired and leading to sugar cravings and overeating.

Complex carbohydrates like whole grains take longer to break down in your body. During processing, whole grains are left intact—the bran, germ, and endosperm are maintained—unlike with white grains where these are removed. Brown rice and whole-wheat flours are considered complex carbs. Other foods found in nature such as sweet potato, fruits, and veggies are also complex carbohydrates. These items contain fiber, which helps keep your little one full and promotes regular bowel movements. They also tend to contain more vitamins and minerals such as magnesium, iron, and folate and protein.

Preventing and Taming Picky Eaters

At this stage it's normal for toddlers to become selective about what they'll eat. But first, know that opinions don't necessarily mean picky eating! We all have opinions about what we eat and that's okay. We consider children to be picky when they start to reject foods they used to enjoy, reducing the number of foods they will eat. When this happens, it is so important to stay strong. And remember, you are the parent! It is your job to provide structured, healthy family meals and snacks. Your child, though, is in charge of how much they eat. I know how frustrating it is and how easy it would be to simply prepare (or heat up) their favorite foods every night but the hard work you put in now will pay off in the future—trust me! Here is your playbook for getting them to eat (period) and eat healthy to boot.

WHY ARE TODDLERS NOTORIOUSLY PICKY EATERS?

It is completely normal for toddlers to go through phases of being disinterested in food and there are a number of reasons for this. This disinterest or "pickiness" can often be more about other things going on with their development. Mainly, it can be more about wanting control than actual pickiness. So much of a toddler's days are filled with adults telling them what to do, but eating is an area where they can really take control. At this age, they also are testing limits. What happens if I throw my plate on the floor even when Mommy told me "no"? And if they are anything like my son, they may just want to play more than they want to do anything else (including sleep). Some kids are still teething which can cause discomfort leading them to want more soft and mushy foods. Teething may cause an overall disinterest in food because eating hurts, but they can't express that. Additionally, after the first 12 months, their growth slows down so they really might just be less hungry.

Speaking of hunger, rule out hunger's main saboteur: too many snacks. Often times kids are given too much in their midmorning or afternoon snack so they really aren't very hungry when they sit down to meals. If your toddler is having milk and food as a snack but doesn't eat their meal, they may just need the food and not the milk. Also, remember a toddler portion is ¼ to ½ cup for each meal and snack. When you actually put that into a measuring cup it may be a lot less than what you might expect. Put another way, that's just 4 to 8 tablespoons worth of food. At the next meal, put all the food for your toddler's meal to the measurement test and see if your expectations of what they might eat match this reality.

Continued on page 46

This is a sample weekly menu I put together using recipes from this book. You can follow this menu when you are just getting started, and as you gain confidence and discover your family's favorite

	MONDAY	TUESDAY	WEDNESDAY
BREAKFAST	Avocado Toast Toads in a Hole (page 93)	½ cup Yogurt, Fruit, and Seed Bowl (page 84)	1 cup Beet Berry Smoothie (page 81)
SNACK	½ sliced apple and 1 tablespoon nut butter	1 to 2 Pumpkin Energy Balls (page 108)	5 to 7 Carrot Fries with 2 tablespoons Citrus-Tahini Dipping Sauce (page 104)
LUNCH	½ to 1 cup White Bean and Kale Soup (page 125)	Salmon and Avocado Salad (page 121)	½ cup Quinoa with Spinach (page 118)
SNACK	1 to 2 Mini Carrot Pancakes (page 58)	⅓ cup edamame	1 to 2 Cacao Sun Butter Bites (page 65)
DINNER	1½ to 3 ounces Maple and Soy Salmon (page 168) and ¼ to ½ cup Cauliflower Rice (page 144)	½ to ¾ cup Mac 'n' Cheese 'n' Peas (page 165) and ¼ cup Roasted Asparagus Tips (page 149)	2 to 4 Almond-Crusted Chicken Fingers (page 175), ¼ cup Beet Applesauce (page 103), and Sweet Potato Bites with Maple-Ginger Dip (page 59)

recipes, you can make your own menu. By taking the time to plan your meals, you will save both time and money at the grocery store and in the kitchen.

THURSDAY	FRIDAY	SATURDAY	SUNDAY
½ to ¾ cup Apple Breakfast Quinoa (page 89)	1 cup Chocolate and Avocado Smoothie with Pepitas (page 80)	2 to 4 Mini Carrot Pancakes (page 58) and ⅓ cup berries	1 to 2 Egg and Spinach Cakes with Feta (page 94)
¼ to ½ cup berries plus Yogurt Cacao Dip (page 67) or 1 string cheese	1 Mini Zucchini Muffin (page 64) or Pumpkin Muffin Mini (page 106)	½ cup whole-milk plain yogurt and 1 tablespoon granola	Roasted Pear Bites (page 68)
Rainbow Pepper Crustless Mini Quiches (page 140) and raw veggies with 1 tablespoon hummus	Tuna Avocado Wraps (page 128)	1 Egg and Spinach Cake with Feta (page 94) and 1 clementine	½ to ¾ cup leftover Turkey Chili (page 180) and ¼ mashed avocado
½ cup Beet Applesauce (page 103)	1 Rainbow Pepper Crustless Mini Quiche (page 140)	1 Mini Zucchini Muffin (page 64) or Pumpkin Muffin Mini (page 106)	½ cup Kale Chips (page 115)
Family Taco Night (page 181)	½ to ¾ cup Turkey Chili (page 180) and 1 cup Kale Chips (page 115)	1½ to 3 ounces Parchment Cod with Veggies (page 167)	1 Veggie Burger with Homemade Ketchup (page 141) and 5 to 7 Carrot Fries with Citrus-Tahini Dipping Sauce (page 104)

Continued from page 43

It's also not such a bad thing for a child to be cautious about new foods that smell or look different. We are cautious as adults and it's a natural instinct. As frustrating as it is in the moment, it's important to know the many reasons why your little one may go through this fussiness stage. They are trying to figure so many things out. The key is to keep offering a variety food of but with little pressure. The more you push, the more he may reject the food. I know firsthand! I had to change my mindset. I let my son know he didn't have to eat it and it wasn't a problem, but he did need to stay seated while Mom and Dad finished their food.

Fussiness around food is a phase, keep offering the nutritious foods, and don't force the issue. Let mealtime still be low-key (as much as possible with a toddler) and they will turn around and surprise you by suddenly eating foods they once rejected. Even showing interest is a big step.

TIPS FOR TAMING PICKINESS

Now we know that pickiness is common. And that we need to trust our children to eat. It's perfectly normal for him to eat a lot one day, and just a little the next. What she enjoys one week, she will flat out reject the next. So, with this knowledge, we can try to relax a bit around meals and enjoy each other's company, without pressuring our little ones to eat more or less. Just focus on your plate. Know you are doing your job by offering healthy foods and sitting at the table together.

Having said that, there are certainly FUN things you can do to get kids more interested in food! Below are some tips and strategies. And no matter what, keep trying. I know how easy it is to get into a rut. I've been there! Here are some tips to inspire you.

ALWAYS HAVE A SAFE FOOD: At mealtimes, include a safe, well-liked food so there is at least one item you know they will love. For example, my son can eat broccoli and grapes all the time so I ensure those are present in addition to the new foods I may introduce.

MAKE MEALS STRUCTURED AND WELL-ROUNDED: Kids like routines so try to have dinner at a similar time each night. We sit in the same seats and I often like to start with some veggies and dip. If he doesn't have his water, he calls me out on it!

BE A ROLE MODEL: My son is always looking at our plates and is very interested in what Mom and Dad are eating. If you want your child to eat more veggies, you've got to eat them too. If you want him to sit down and eat, you better have your meals seated (my husband and I are always reminding each other to do that and just not shovel food in while standing in the kitchen). My son often asks "Mommy likes X?" I say "yes, do you want to try?" He may say "yes" (and may subsequently spit it out) or "no," but either way it's his choice.

MAKE THE DINNER TABLE STRESS-FREE: We are huge fans of playing music at the dinner table whether it be toddler radio, jazz, or adult songs. My son loves music and I know it puts him in a good mood.

PRESENTATION HELPS: The amount of time I have spent searching for fun dinnerware, utensils, and cookie cutters (see page 15) is absurd but it does help in making mealtime fun!

LET THEM CHOOSE THEIR PACE: I am a fast eater but often remind myself that kids are so good about eating at their own speed and getting what they need (unless distracted by something). So, I have to pace myself and understand that my son may take a 10-minute break between bites and that's okay.

GIVE THEM SOME CHOICE: Offer them two veggie options. Do you want broccoli or asparagus? Should I bake it or steam it? It's giving your child some control, but not in an overwhelming way. And they will feel like they made the decision about what to eat.

TALK ABOUT FOOD AWAY FROM THE TABLE: I am a huge supporter of reading books on food, getting veggie temporary tattoos (from Tater Tats), and even subscribing to the veggie of the month club (from Veggie Buds Club). Non-mealtimes are less high stakes and encourage increased curiosity.

TRY A DIP: My son loves to dip all foods! We have included four fun dips, the Citrus-Tahini Dipping Sauce (page 104), Zucchini Dip (page 111), Lemon-Yogurt Dipping Sauce (page 166), and

Avocado Dipping Sauce (page 112) in this cookbook, as well as a recipe for Homemade Ketchup (page 141). Commercially bought (or homemade) salad dressings and hummus also work beautifully.

GET THEM IN THE KITCHEN: During our morning routine making smoothies, Julian loves to scoop various seeds and now he says "I need my hemp hearts!" It's so cute. I let him pick a few ingredients. When we cook together, he typically likes to sample what we make. At times, he may spit it out and say "I don't like that" and other times he may say "yummy." Either way, he is game to try on his own terms so I find that a win.

BRING THEM TO THE FARMERS' MARKET: I always ask Julian what two items he wants to pick at the farmers' market. Do whatever you can do to encourage participation, independence, and interest! Julian also loves to grocery shop. He has his own little cart and likes to pick what we need. We start in the produce section and I let him grab stuff even if it wasn't originally on my shopping list.

TEACH THEM ABOUT THE HEALTH BENEFITS OF CERTAIN FOODS: For example, I told my son that carrots are good for his eyes so he can see better. Once he takes a bite, it gets digested by his tummy, and then goes to his eyes. He was fascinated.

Do these tips work all the time? No, but they do certainly help, are fun (rather than nagging or bribing), and they help develop a curiosity and understanding of where food comes from.

TRY AND TRY AGAIN, 10 TO 15 TIMES

When I first heard the advice to try a food 10 to 15 times or even 15 to 20 times, I thought "oh wow, that's a lot of work!" But here's the thing, it does actually work. You don't need to be super precise about it either. Meaning it doesn't need to be every day for 10 days, but within a week or a few months expose your child to a variety of foods. Try to aim for a new food (or a food item your child doesn't normally eat) every day if possible. When introducing a new food, I recommend offering a small amount, starting with just a taste at first. Let them explore the food on their own. After about 10 attempts, if it's a no-go then try getting creative. You can cut the food into different shapes, try different plates, a dip, or even try offering it in a new location (like a picnic in the park). Have your little one help prepare it or even help plate the food. Most importantly don't force them to try. It will only backfire. And remember, toddlers don't like all foods just like you, so be prepared for them to reject a food altogether. That's completely normal.

YOUR TODDLER EATING QUESTIONS ANSWERED

My toddler only likes white food. Are they getting enough protein?

I get this question all the time. Even though I do emphasize that your toddler has a protein with every meal and ideally in at least one of her snacks, it's actually not that difficult for them to meet their protein needs. Toddlers need roughly 13 to 16 grams of protein a day and odds are your toddler is getting that.

For example, below are some common foods and how much protein they contain in just one serving:

* 1 egg = 6 grams of protein
* 1 cup yogurt = 8 grams of protein
* ¼ cup beans = 3 grams of protein
* 1 ounce chicken = 7 grams of protein
* 1 tablespoon nut butter = 4 grams of protein
* ¼ cup cooked quinoa = 2 grams of protein
* 3 tablespoons hemp hearts = 10 grams of protein
* 1 sprouted bread slice = 4 grams of protein
* ¼ cup whole-wheat flour = 4 grams of protein
* ¼ cup oats = 3½ grams of protein
* ¼ cup dry brown rice = 4 grams of protein

My toddler doesn't like to sit at the table longer than 5 minutes and would prefer to graze while playing. What should I do?

I feel for you and I definitely struggled with this with Julian. He would not sit still and dinner time felt like a battle. I was always so envious of those kids I saw at restaurants who sat pleasantly for the entire meal when we were up and out of our seats entertaining our son. For your active toddler, having them sit down for a 30-minute dinner may not be realistic, but get them to understand that your family sits down at a table for meals. You can certainly try building up the time. So, start with five minutes first, then the following week aim for eight minutes and keep building from there. You can set a timer or use a clock if that appeals to your toddler. Try to limit distractions at the table and most importantly be sure to sit down with your toddler and participate in the meal with them.

You want to avoid grazing all day and focus on sitting down for designated meals and snacks. The goal is to have your toddler hungry come mealtime, and constantly grazing interferes with

MORE ON KIDS IN THE KITCHEN

Eating is a sensory experience. Food should be touched, smelled, seen, and tasted. When children participate in preparing food, they are more likely to try it (ahem: vegetables). Do this as much as possible to keep them engaged and curious. Kids love being sous chefs! Purchase an apron and, if they will wear it, a chef's hat, and get them some kid-friendly kitchen supplies.

A child-safe knife and a child-size apron can go a long way. Focus more on the food prep than the final product. Emphasize the fun in purchasing and making the food rather than tasting the food.

Give your little ones simple, reduced-mess tasks throughout the cooking process:

* Tear kale and lettuce with fingers
* Place fruits like bananas and avocados (good for pancakes, muffins, and guacamole recipes) in a sealed bag and encourage kids to mash it up with their hands and fists
* Have children roll citrus fruits on the counter using their palms to soften the rind which helps better release the juice
* Pour liquids
* Stir batters
* Add ingredients to a blender and turn it on and off
* Pick herbs off stems
* Wash produce
* Grease baking pans

that. Another tip: Keep beverages to between meals so they don't fill up on liquids!

My toddler loves pasta sauce. Can I just purée all veggies he needs into the sauce?

The key here is to have your kids learn, taste, and explore different foods, tastes, and textures. It is so tempting to just hide (or fortify) nutritious foods in other foods like sauces from time to time, but you also want your child to recognize and enjoy these foods on their own. I am all for incorporating a variety of vegetables into recipes just as you would any other nutrient-rich food, but don't use it as a crutch—keep introducing vegetables in other forms as well.

My toddler still likes to be spoon-fed. Can't I just feed her? It's so much less messy.

Self-feeding is incredibly important and allowing your child to decide what they consume will benefit them in the long term, as it allows them to explore textures and flavors and, most importantly, go at their own pace. And the mess will decrease as they get older!

My son can't tolerate cow's milk. Can I give him nut milk instead?

You can certainly introduce nuts and seeds at this point, but while nuts and seeds are a good source of protein and fiber, the liquid made from them (particularly those you purchase at a store) contains very little of either. I recommend adding a protein and fat source to what you are using it with, for example, a smoothie or as a base for oatmeal. If choosing nut milk, find ones that don't use carrageenan (a preservative used as a thickening agent and stabilizer). Choose the unsweetened version and rotate between the various options. Ideally, try making your own (see pages 76 and 77). They are very easy and much more nutritious when made at home. For a natural sweetener, I recommend using dates, pure maple syrup, or raw honey (if your child is over 12 months old).

Is drinking cow's milk essential for healthy bones?

Many people worry that if they don't consume dairy they will be missing out on calcium to support their growing bones. What we know is that calcium is not the only nutrient needed for bone health. The body needs a combination of nutrients, like vitamin D, magnesium, and vitamin K. Also, dairy isn't the only way to get calcium. There are many other great sources from the foods we eat, like green leafy veggies (think kale, collard greens, broccoli, and bok choy), sesame seeds, edamame, white beans, chickpeas and oranges. So if milk doesn't agree with your child, there are other ways to meet their needs for peak bone health.

Help, my toddler is constipated! What should I do?

Potty talk, I love it! Constipation can be very common in kids. A combination of food choices, drinking habits (or lack thereof), medications, travel, potty behaviors like withholding, and inefficient posture can all be culprits. Apart from being uncomfortable, this can lead to a reduced appetite. Additionally, poop is the one way that your kiddo can eliminate toxins from their body which can have a direct impact on their mood! I always find that my son is much happier and hungry right after a big poop. (He will be so embarrassed to see this in print one day!)

But what is true constipation? If your child skips a poop one day, it doesn't mean he is constipated. Normal is different for each child. The definition of constipation in kids is a change in the regular bowel habits along with stools that are difficult to pass. Usually the not-so-fun symptoms like bellyaches and gas accompany it. So, if your child always goes every other day and is symptom-free, they are not necessarily constipated.

The good news is that there are things you can do to speed up those sluggish guts. Below are some tips to get things moving!

HYDRATE: Water is number one when it comes to managing bowel movements! So, have them drink up. Find what works best for your child. Sometimes they prefer straws, other times they prefer to drink out of "Mommy's cup," or a new cup. Sometimes I play a game of cheers and that gets my son drinking as he can literally play "cheers" 20 times! Drinking water is just as important as fiber when managing constipation.

Bumping up the fiber without increasing fluid can actually make things worse!

UP THE FIBER: Increase fiber in your child's diet by adding these favorite fiber boosters:

GROUND FLAXSEED: Add to yogurt, oatmeal, or muffins. Or make it into a flax pancake by grinding 1 to 2 tablespoons flaxseed (or purchase ground flaxseed) and mix with an egg yolk. Cook in grass-fed butter or coconut oil.

LEGUMES, FRUITS, AND VEGGIES : Increase offerings of these fiber-rich foods.

DRIED FRUIT LIKE PRUNES, DATES, FIGS, AND APRICOTS (START WITH 2): Hydrate in boiling water until plump and then purée. You can add this to any yogurt or oatmeal, or give it to them straight up.

REDUCE THESE FOODS: Foods to consider reducing as they can be binding if the problem is consistent:

* Dairy products
* Cereal fortified with iron or any iron supplements you may be using
* White rice
* White flour foods
* Rice cereal

PROBIOTICS: These are essential for proper digestion. They are naturally found in fermented foods like pickles, yogurt, and kefir and are great for regulation. You can also start them on a daily probiotic. It can make a huge difference.

THE FAMILY THAT EATS TOGETHER

From day one you need to set your priorities. Mine were to spend as much time with my family, and not in the kitchen, as possible. To do that, I had to commit to preparing one meal for the whole family and not taking everyone's personal order. I know, it's hard but if you set that goal early, you can achieve it. For example, very early on, my husband and I would blend up our adult dinners into a purée for Julian. That way we spent less time preparing and more time together. Plus, our son was exposed to a wide variety of different flavors, textures, and nutrients from the start. He learned to like "difficult" flavors early on and as he transitioned to whole foods, those tastes remained, though with a different texture. Now as Julian is older, I make a real effort to make just one dinner for all of us. He doesn't always love what we put in front of him, but again we ensure there is always one thing that we know he likes as part of our meal. That way if dinner bombs, he's still getting in something nutritious.

I take the same approach with veggies. Early on we blended all different combinations to challenge his palate in preparation for whole foods (think spinach, rutabaga, and onion). Now that he's eating fully composed meals those flavors are still in his memory bank. He doesn't love everything he used to eat; many times that's due to texture (leafy foods are harder for toddlers to wrap their heads and mouths around). But we ensure that he always sees vegetables, and more importantly sees Mom and Dad eating vegetables. At every meal, we bring out some hummus and baby carrots, radishes, celery, or cucumbers, things that are easy to grab. He sees us eating them so he gets curious! You can also get creative. We've made kale chips, veggie dips, and soups—the sky is the limit. This book is filled with loads of veggie ideas to get you started.

This Book's Recipes

Now on to the fun part! These recipes are a combination of my family's, friends', and clients' favorites. They are meant to be first and foremost nutritious but also EASY. The majority of the recipes can be made in under 30 minutes which is key. As I have learned and experienced as a working mom with a toddler, you can have all the tools and knowledge about nutrition but unless it is realistic, it's not going to happen, or it may happen at the cost of a lot of added stress. The recipes in this book:

1. Are made with nutritious, whole ingredients
2. Are meant for the whole family including toddler, older kids, and adults
3. Are tasty, balanced meals
4. Can often be made in 30 minutes or less
5. Can often be made ahead of time and frozen or made in bulk

6. Might have an option to make in the slow cooker—add the ingredients in the morning and by evening it is all done
7. Are made with antioxidants and nourishing foods to set your family up for a healthy future
8. Are gut friendly
9. Are made with full-fat ingredients, nothing low-fat
10. Are made with only the best sources of sugar, nothing refined

Colorful labels ensure you'll also know if the recipe conforms to your dietary restrictions. Here's what you'll see:

DF Dairy Free
GF Gluten Free
NF Nut Free
V   Vegetarian
Vegan Vegan (of course!)

There is so much information and I know I had to really do a lot of research for my son at this stage, even though I am a dietitian! Information is constantly evolving so this book is an accumulation of my knowledge as a dietitian and tried-and-true strategies as a mom. I hope your family enjoys them as much as we do!

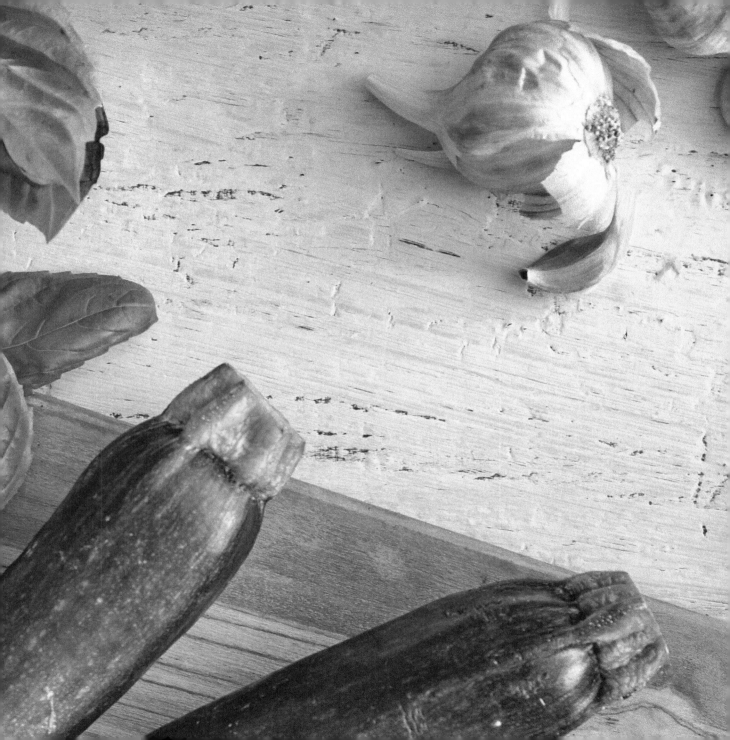

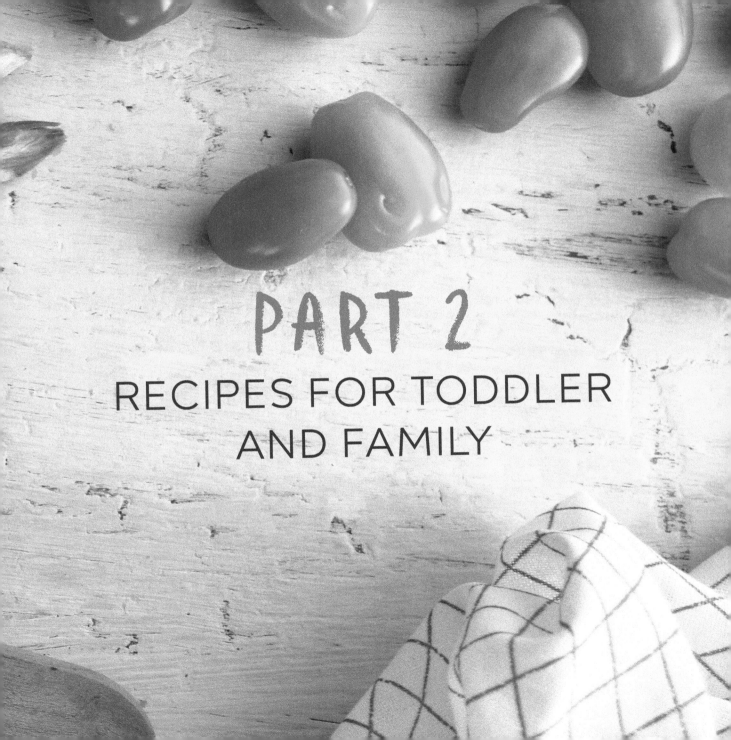

PART 2
RECIPES FOR TODDLER AND FAMILY

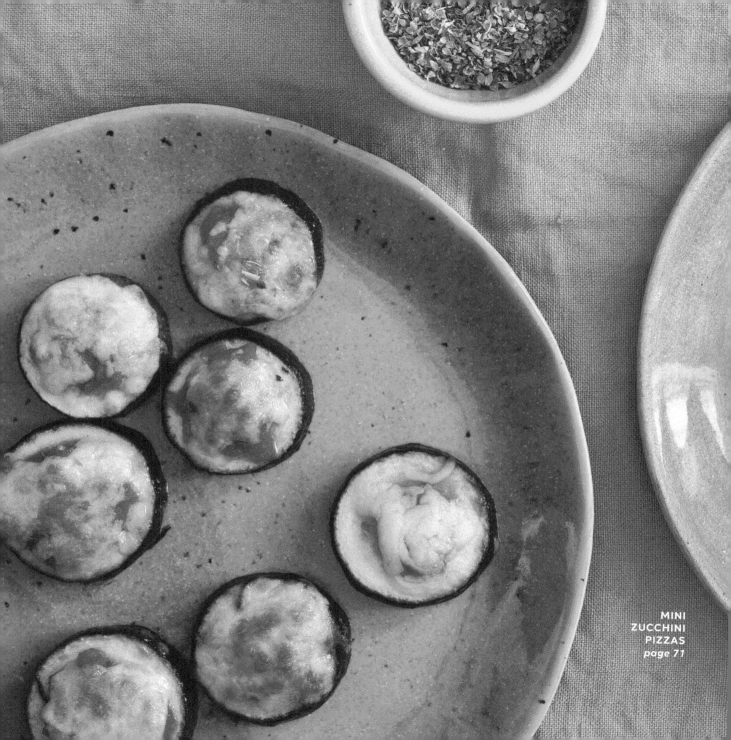

MINI
ZUCCHINI
PIZZAS
page 71

4

FINGER FOODS

Finger foods are the first foods your toddler eats as he or she starts to incorporate more solid foods with the purées, generally between the ages of 9 and 12 months. These finger foods will certainly work for older toddlers and preschoolers as well (I have been known to snack on them too!), but these recipes are designed specifically for very young toddlers who are just starting this next step in their solid food journey. These foods are soft enough that they are not a choking hazard, but they have enough chew that your toddler will get experience with chewing foods. They also don't have ingredients that are problematic for younger toddlers, like honey. They're perfect for snacks or as part of your toddler's favorite meals.

Mini Carrot Pancakes

NF V

SERVES 4

PREP TIME: 5 MINUTES
COOK TIME: 15 MINUTES

1 cup whole-wheat flour

1 teaspoon
baking powder

½ teaspoon baking soda

Pinch kosher salt

½ teaspoon
ground ginger

½ teaspoon ground
cinnamon

1 large egg, beaten

1 cup whole milk or
buttermilk

1½ cups grated carrots

Butter or oil, for cooking

You can freeze and reheat these small pancakes, so they're great to make ahead in a big batch and pull out when you need a quick snack. Reheat two pancakes in the microwave, about 30 seconds to 1 minute for thawed or 90 seconds to 2 minutes for frozen. For very young toddlers, you may want to cut these up into smaller pieces.

1. In a medium bowl, whisk together the flour, baking powder, baking soda, salt, ginger, and cinnamon.
2. In a small bowl, whisk together the egg and milk.
3. Add the wet ingredients to the dry and mix until just combined; streaks of flour will remain in the batter.
4. Fold in the carrots until just combined.
5. Heat a nonstick skillet on medium-high heat. Oil the pan with a small amount of oil or butter, swirling to coat.
6. Using a heaping tablespoon, drop the batter into rounds on the preheated skillet. Cook for about 3 minutes, until bubbles form on the surface of the pancake. Flip and cook for 2 to 3 minutes more, until cooked through.

SUBSTITUTION TIP: Make this dairy-free by replacing the buttermilk with an equal amount of nondairy milk. To make it gluten-free, replace the whole-wheat flour with buckwheat flour or another whole-grain, gluten-free flour.

Sweet Potato Bites with Maple-Ginger Dip

SERVES 4 TO 6

PREP TIME: 5 MINUTES
COOK TIME: 20 MINUTES

1 sweet potato, peeled
and cut into ¼- to
½-inch pieces

1 tablespoon extra-virgin
olive oil

½ cup plain whole-
milk yogurt

1 tablespoon pure
maple syrup

½ teaspoon fresh
ginger, grated

Sweet potatoes have an earthy sweetness that kids enjoy. They are a great source of vitamins and fiber, including vitamins A, C, and E. This recipe also harnesses kids' love of dipping with a slightly sweet but healthy dip. Allow the sweet potatoes to cool slightly (or completely) before you give them to your toddler. You can also freeze them in ½- to 1-cup serving sizes in individual ziptop bags, toss into your bag frozen, and allow to thaw for an on-the-go snack without the dip.

1. Preheat the oven to 375°F and line a baking sheet with parchment paper.
2. In a medium bowl, toss the sweet potatoes and olive oil. Transfer the sweet potatoes in a single layer to the prepared baking sheet.
3. Cook for 15 to 20 minutes, until they begin to brown. Remove from the oven and cool slightly.
4. While the sweet potatoes are cooling, in a small bowl, whisk together the yogurt, maple syrup, and ginger. Serve as a dip with the sweet potatoes.

SUBSTITUTION TIP: To make this vegan and dairy-free, replace the yogurt with coconut or almond milk yogurt.

Mini Frozen Yogurt-Berry Bites

GF NF V

SERVES 6

PREP TIME: 5 MINUTES,
PLUS 3 TO 6 HOURS
FREEZING TIME

1 cup plain whole-
milk yogurt

1 cup fresh or frozen
berries (strawberries,
raspberries, blueberries,
blackberries, or a mix)

These snacks are about as simple as it gets, and they have a sweet, creamy flavor. They're also an excellent source of calcium and were one of my favorite simple snacks when Julian was just starting finger foods. They are easy to make ahead in large batches on the weekend and then freeze in single-serving containers until you're ready to use them. No thawing necessary.

1. Line a baking sheet with parchment paper.
2. In a blender or food processor (or in a bowl if using an immersion blender), combine the yogurt and berries. Process until smooth.
3. Drop by ⅛ teaspoons onto the baking sheet.
4. Freeze for 3 to 6 hours.
5. Store in a tightly sealed container. These will safely store in the freezer for about 3 months.

SUBSTITUTION TIP: To make this vegan and dairy-free, replace the yogurt with coconut or almond milk yogurt. You can also vary the berries with other soft fruits, such as bananas or peeled peaches.

Celery Root and Sweet Potato Cakes

SERVES 8

PREP TIME: 5 MINUTES
COOK TIME: 12 MINUTES

½ cup peeled and grated celery root

½ cup sweet potato, peeled and grated

½ teaspoon ground cumin

1 large egg, beaten

1 tablespoon extra-virgin olive oil plus 1 teaspoon, divided

Kosher salt (optional)

Celery root, also known as celeriac, is a mild, earthy root vegetable you can find in most grocery stores. It's an excellent source of fiber, vitamin K, and vitamin B$_6$, while sweet potatoes add sweetness and vitamins A, C, and E. These freeze well (up to three months), and you can reheat them in a 350°F oven for about 5 minutes or serve them cold. They are delicious alone or with my favorite Beet Applesauce (page 103) recipe.

1. In a large bowl, combine the celery root, sweet potato, cumin, egg, and 1 tablespoon olive oil, mixing until well combined.
2. Heat a large, nonstick skillet on medium-high heat. Brush the bottom of the pan with the remaining 1 teaspoon of olive oil.
3. Form 2-tablespoon cakes, and put them in the preheated pan, flattening them slightly with the spatula.
4. Cook for 3 to 4 minutes per side, flipping once, until golden brown.
5. Season with salt (if using).

SUBSTITUTION TIP: If you can't find celery root, you can replace it with an equal amount of another grated root vegetable, such as parsnip, daikon radish, or carrot.

PREP TIP: Use the grater attachment on your food processor for quick grating.

Cauliflower Tots

NF V

SERVES 8

PREP TIME: 15 MINUTES
COOK TIME: 45 MINUTES

1 cauliflower head,
cut from the stalk and
broken into florets

¼ cup Parmesan
cheese, grated

1 large egg, beaten

¼ cup whole-wheat
bread crumbs

½ teaspoon garlic powder

½ teaspoon
onion powder

Kosher salt (optional)

Replacing potato with cauliflower reduces starch and adds more fiber and vitamin C than potatoes. These cauliflower tots take about 45 minutes in the oven, but it's passive time, so you can play with your kiddo while they cook. The active time is only about 15 minutes, and the tots make a delicious snack. You can refrigerate or freeze and reheat them in the microwave or in a 350°F oven for about 20 minutes.

1. Preheat the oven to 350°F. Line a baking sheet with parchment paper.
2. Bring a large pot of water to a boil and add the cauliflower florets. Cook, covered, until they are tender, about 10 minutes. Drain in a colander.
3. Add the cauliflower to a food processor and pulse for 10 (1-second) pulses, until it resembles rice.
4. In a large bowl, combine the cauliflower with the cheese, egg, bread crumbs, garlic powder, and onion powder. Working 1 tablespoon at a time, form the mixture into tater tot–shaped pieces. Arrange in a single layer on the prepared baking sheet.
5. Bake for 45 minutes, flipping once, until browned and cooked through.

SUBSTITUTION TIP: For gluten-free, replace the bread crumbs with gluten-free whole-grain bread crumbs. To make your own gluten-free bread crumbs, simply remove the crusts from whole-grain gluten-free sandwich bread and pulse it in the food processor for 10 to 20 (1-second) pulses.

Mini Spinach Cheese Bites

SERVES 6

PREP TIME: 15 MINUTES
COOK TIME: 15 MINUTES

½ cup frozen chopped
spinach, defrosted and
wrung of excess water
(use a tea towel and
wring over the sink)

1 large egg, beaten

¼ cup Cheddar
cheese, grated

1 teaspoon dried thyme

¾ cup cooked brown rice

1 teaspoon garlic powder

¼ teaspoon kosher salt

To make these super easy little bites of goodness, buy precooked brown rice or precook the rice yourself and save it in 1-cup servings in your freezer for up to 6 months. These bites taste great cold too, so all you need to do is thaw them. For younger toddlers, cut the balls into fourths before serving.

1. Preheat the oven to 350°F. Line a baking sheet with parchment paper.
2. In a large bowl, combine the spinach, egg, cheese, thyme, brown rice, garlic powder, and salt, mixing well.
3. Form into 1-tablespoon balls and place them on the prepared baking sheet.
4. Bake for 15 to 20 minutes, until browned.

SUBSTITUTION TIP: You can make these dairy-free by using any nondairy, vegan cheese in place of the Cheddar cheese.

Mini Zucchini Muffins

NF V

SERVES 12

PREP TIME: 15 MINUTES
COOK TIME: 15 MINUTES

1 teaspoon coconut oil

1¾ cups whole-wheat flour

1 teaspoon baking powder

½ teaspoon baking soda

1 teaspoon ground cinnamon

Pinch kosher salt

¼ cup extra-virgin olive oil

¼ cup pure maple syrup

2 large eggs

1 cup buttermilk

1½ cups grated zucchini

Mini muffins are a parent's best friend. This recipe is forgiving and extremely versatile. You can customize it to your toddler's current tastes. For example, if your tot doesn't love zucchini, replace it with grated carrots or grated butternut squash and switch out the spices, such as using savory spices like cumin and coriander. These freeze well in resealable plastic bags (up to 6 months), and they thaw quickly due to their small size, so healthy snacks are always only a few minutes away.

1. Preheat the oven to 400°F. Brush a 12-cup mini muffin tin with coconut oil.
2. In a large bowl, whisk together the wheat flour, baking powder, baking soda, cinnamon, and salt.
3. In a small bowl, whisk together the olive oil, maple syrup, eggs, and buttermilk.
4. Add the wet ingredients to the dry ingredients, mixing until just combined. Streaks of flour will remain in the batter.
5. Fold in the zucchini.
6. Spoon the batter into the prepared muffin tin.
7. Bake for 15 minutes, until the muffins are golden and a toothpick inserted in the center comes out clean. Cool on a rack before serving.

SUBSTITUTION TIP: For children over 12 months, you can replace the maple syrup with honey, if desired.

Cacao Sun Butter Bites

SERVES 10

PREP TIME: 15 MINUTES

¼ cup coconut flour

¼ cup unsweetened cacao powder

⅓ cup sun butter

1 to 2 tablespoons pure maple syrup

¼ cup milk or nondairy milk (see page 76 and 77)

These little bites freeze well in a resealable plastic bag. They are creamy and chocolatey with a lightly sweet flavor—something your toddler will love. For younger toddlers or if you worry about choking, cut each bite into quarters.

1. In a medium bowl, combine the coconut flour, cacao powder, sun butter, and maple syrup, creaming ingredients together to mix well.
2. Slowly add the milk, stirring, until the texture is similar to cookie dough and can easily be formed into balls.
3. Form into 1-tablespoon balls and refrigerate or freeze until you are ready to serve them.

SUBSTITUTION TIP: For children over 12 months, you can replace the maple syrup with honey, if desired. To make these bites vegan, use a nondairy milk like coconut milk or oat milk.

Roasted Butternut Squash and Thyme Bites

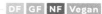

SERVES 4

PREP TIME: 10 MINUTES
COOK TIME: 20 MINUTES

1 cup butternut squash, cut into ¼- to ½-inch pieces

1 tablespoon extra-virgin olive oil

1 teaspoon dried thyme

¼ teaspoon kosher salt

Many grocery stores now sell pre-cut butternut squash, which is a time-saver. For younger toddlers, you may still want to cut pre-cut squash cubes in half before baking to minimize choking hazards. These will freeze well for up to 3 months.

1. Preheat the oven to 400°F.
2. In a small bowl, toss the squash with olive oil and thyme. Spread in a single layer on a rimmed baking sheet.
3. Bake for 15 to 20 minutes, until the squash is tender and starts to brown.
4. Season with salt and serve.

SUBSTITUTION TIP: Acorn or delicata squash or pumpkin works well here too.

Yogurt Cacao Dip with Berries

SERVES 2

PREP TIME: 10 MINUTES

½ cup plain whole-milk yogurt

2 teaspoons unsweetened cacao powder

1 tablespoon pure maple syrup

1 cup strawberries, sliced

Toddlers love to explore their food with their hands, and eating is a great sensory learning opportunity. This is why dip is such a fun (but messy) option with your kiddos. Put down a splat mat, give your toddler this tasty dip, and offer him some sliced strawberries to dip into it. He'll love the flavor and the experience. The dip will store in the fridge for up to 3 days.

1. In a small bowl, whisk together the yogurt, cacao powder, and maple syrup.
2. Serve with the strawberries for dipping.

SUBSTITUTION TIP: To make this vegan, you can use a plain yogurt made from coconut milk or almond milk.

INGREDIENT TIP: Cacao powder is a less-processed form of cacao beans made by cold-pressing unroasted cocoa beans. Cocoa powder is made by roasting the cacao at high temperatures, therefore reducing the nutritional value of the cacao. When possible, use cacao instead of cocoa, but if you can't find cacao, cocoa powder will work fine in these recipes.

Roasted Pear Bites

DF GF NF Vegan

SERVES 2 TO 4

PREP TIME: 10 MINUTES
COOK TIME: 20 MINUTES

1 pear, peeled, cored and cut into ½-inch cubes

½ teaspoon ground cinnamon

Roasting pears softens them and brings out their sweet, mellow flavor. It's also a great way to add some spice to the pears, which brings out their natural sweetness without having to add extra sugar. These are great as a finger food, or you can add them to yogurt for a quick snack.

1. Preheat the oven to 425°F.
2. On a nonstick rimmed baking sheet, arrange the pears in a single layer. Sprinkle with the cinnamon.
3. Bake for about 20 minutes, turning once, until the pears begin to brown.

SUBSTITUTION TIP: This works well with apples, too. You can also vary the spices, replacing the cinnamon with an equal amount of ground ginger, allspice, or a mix of cloves and nutmeg.

Baked Zucchini and Carrot Fritters

NF V

SERVES 2 TO 4

PREP TIME: 10 MINUTES
COOK TIME: 20 MINUTES

1 zucchini, grated
(about 1 cup)

2 carrots, grated
(about 1 cup)

3 scallions, both white
and green parts,
thinly sliced

2 large eggs, beaten

½ cup Cheddar or
Parmesan cheese, grated

¼ cup whole-wheat flour

¼ teaspoon kosher salt

The key to these fritters is removing as much moisture as possible from the vegetables so they don't wind up soggy. To do this, put the grated veggies in a colander in the sink, place a plate on top of them, and press on the plate to extrude the water. Or wrap the grated veggies in a tea towel and wring them out over the sink.

1. Preheat the oven to 400°F. Line a baking sheet with parchment paper.
2. In a large bowl, combine the zucchini, carrots, scallions, eggs, cheese, and flour. Using clean hands, mix until well combined.
3. Form the mixture in 2-tablespoon balls, and arrange the balls on the prepared baking sheet, flattening as you do so.
4. Bake for 15 to 20 minutes, flipping once, until browned.
5. Season with salt.

SUBSTITUTION TIP: Other summer squashes such as patty pan make a great substitution for zucchini, and you can replace the carrots with other root veggies, such as parsnips or potatoes.

Soft Scramble with Grated Veggies

SERVES 1

PREP TIME: 10 MINUTES
COOK TIME: 10 MINUTES

1 tablespoon extra-virgin olive oil

¼ cup butternut squash, grated

1 tablespoon red bell pepper, grated or very finely chopped

2 large eggs, beaten

¼ teaspoon kosher salt

If you're looking for a quick protein-rich meal or snack for your toddler, you can't go wrong with scrambling some eggs. The great thing about eggs, beyond their nutritional value, is just how easy it is to customize them to even the pickiest of toddler tastes, and you can make them in about 10 minutes.

1. In a small, nonstick pan, heat the olive oil on medium high until it shimmers.
2. Add the squash and bell pepper and cook about 3 minutes, stirring occasionally, until soft.
3. Add the eggs and scramble for 2 to 3 minutes more, until the eggs are cooked.
4. Season with salt.

SUBSTITUTION TIP: Any grated, small, or finely chopped veggies work here. Some to consider: peas, zucchini, carrots, scallions, or spinach.

Mini Zucchini Pizzas

SERVES 4

PREP TIME: 10 MINUTES
COOK TIME: 10 MINUTES

1 tablespoon avocado oil

1 tablespoon extra-virgin
olive oil

½ small zucchini, cut into
¼-inch-thick rounds

½ cup canned crushed
tomatoes

¼ teaspoon garlic powder

¼ teaspoon
dried oregano

½ cup mozzarella cheese,
finely grated

Kids tend to love pizza and this healthy version is no exception. Perfect for tiny hands, these little pizza bites are a wonderful way to introduce zucchini in a fun form. Have your little one help you assemble them and get in on the fun.

1. Preheat the broiler. Grease a baking sheet with avocado oil.
2. In a large sauté pan, heat the olive oil over medium-high heat until it shimmers.
3. Add the zucchini rounds and cook for about 5 minutes, until softened. Place the zucchini rounds in a single layer on the prepared baking sheet.
4. In a small bowl, combine the tomatoes, garlic powder, and oregano and mix well. Spoon an equal portion of the tomato sauce on each zucchini round and top with an equal portion of the cheese.
5. Broil for about 5 minutes, until the cheese melts. Store remaining mini pizzas in the refrigerator for up to 3 days or in the freezer for up to 6 months.

METHOD TIP: Sometimes zucchini can be a little watery. You can remedy this by simply squeezing the liquid out using a towel.

Warm Black Bean and Avocado Salad

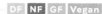

SERVES 4

PREP TIME: 10 MINUTES
COOK TIME: 10 MINUTES

1 tablespoon extra-virgin olive oil

¼ cup diced onion

1 (14-ounce) can black beans, drained

½ teaspoon ground cumin

½ teaspoon dried oregano

½ teaspoon garlic powder

½ teaspoon chili powder (optional)

½ avocado, cut into small cubes

1 tablespoon lime juice (optional)

½ teaspoon kosher salt (optional)

This will keep well in the fridge for up to 3 days, and reheats easily on the stove or in the microwave. Store the beans by themselves and cut up the avocado just before serving for best results.

1. In a small, nonstick pan, heat the olive oil on medium high until it shimmers.
2. Add the onion and cook for about 3 minutes, stirring until soft.
3. Add the black beans, cumin, oregano, and garlic powder. Cook for about 3 minutes, stirring occasionally, until the beans are heated through. Remove a toddler portion.
4. Stir in the chili powder (if using) and cook for 2 minutes more. Remove from the heat.
5. For the toddler portion, sprinkle a few avocado cubes over the salad and serve. Stir the remaining avocado into the pan. Squeeze the lime juice over the top (if using) and season with kosher salt (if using).

INGREDIENT TIP: To cut avocados, cut around the outside lengthwise down to the pit. Then, twist the avocado to separate. Using the half of the avocado without the pit, use a knife to cut the avocados into the desired shape and then scoop out of the peel with a large spoon.

Simple Fruit Salad

SERVES 4

PREP TIME: 10 MINUTES

½ banana, halved lengthwise and sliced

½ cup cantaloupe, cut into ¼- to ½-inch cubes

½ cup raspberries, halved

½ cup peeled pear and cut into ¼- to ½-inch cubes (½ cup)

½ cup watermelon, cut into ¼- to ½-inch cubes

¼ teaspoon ground ginger

Soft fruits make an easy-to-eat and tasty finger-food fruit salad for your toddler. Any soft fruit cut into bite-size pieces will work well here, and this will store for 2 days in the fridge.

In a small bowl, combine the banana, cantaloupe, raspberries, pear, watermelon, and ginger. Mix well.

INGREDIENT TIP: Simple cookie cutters create fun shapes!

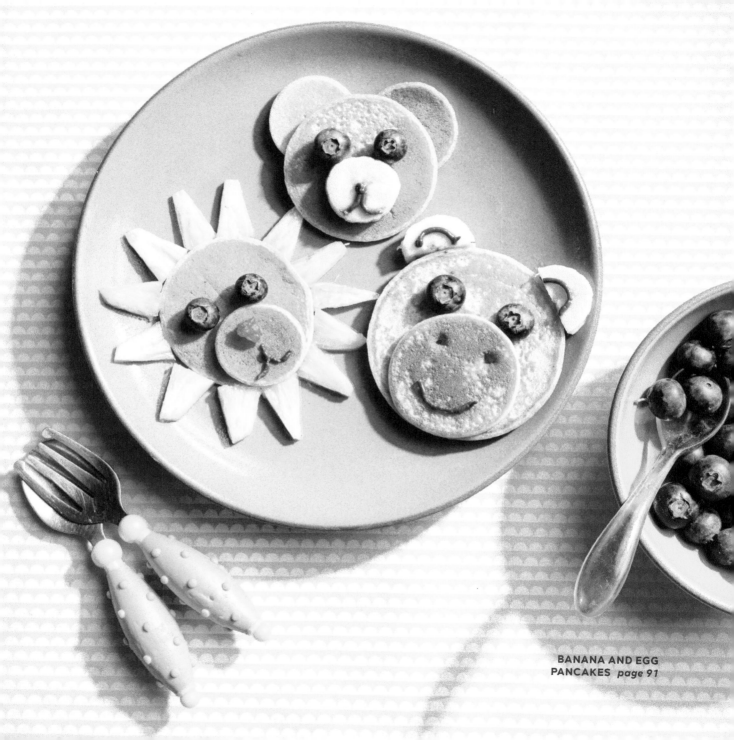

BANANA AND EGG
PANCAKES *page 91*

5

SMOOTHIES AND BREAKFAST

Breakfast is truly my favorite meal of the day. In the recipes that follow, you will find many of the options can be made ahead or made very quickly for those rushed mornings. We enjoy a lot of smoothies in my house, as they make great breakfasts, but they're also good for quick snacks or meals on the go. You can even put smoothies in reusable pouches and your toddler can enjoy them like purées. My favorite make-ahead breakfasts are the Chocolate Chip Oat Banana Blender Muffins (page 92) and the Broccoli and Cheese Mini Frittata Muffins (page 85).

Nutritionally, it's important to include a good source of protein, fat, and some fiber in the form of fruit or veggies at breakfast. If you need to start somewhere to make a difference in your toddler's nutrition, start here! It will make a huge impact on their energy, mood, focus, sleep, and cravings for the rest of the day.

Nondairy Milks

Nondairy milks are so popular these days, and there are a ton of varieties at the supermarket. The problem is that they often contain fillers and preservatives. If you've tried making your own nut or seed milk yourself, you realize not only how easy it is but how much better it actually tastes! You can control the thickness and taste, and they can be flavored many different ways. Below are some simple nut and seed milks to get you started. For creamier milks, soak the nuts overnight.

Cashew Milk

DF | GF | Vegan

MAKES 3 TO 4 CUPS

PREP TIME: 5 MINUTES, PLUS 1 HOUR FOR SOAKING

¾ cup raw unsalted cashews

1 pitted date (optional)

½ teaspoon vanilla extract (optional)

Dash salt (optional)

1. Place raw cashews in a bowl and cover with cold water. Allow to soak for at least 1 hour or as long as overnight, then drain and rinse.
2. In a blender jar, combine the soaked cashews and 3 to 4 cups filtered water.
3. Blend on low, then slowly increase to high for 1 to 2 minutes until the milk is completely smooth.
4. Add the date, vanilla (if using), and/or salt (if using), then blend again to combine. Use immediately, or transfer to an airtight storage container and refrigerate for 4 to 5 days.

METHOD TIP: Cashews get so soft after soaking that they typically don't need to be strained. For a thicker texture, scrape down the sides then blend again for another minute.

Hemp Milk

MAKES 4 CUPS

PREP TIME: 5 MINUTES

½ cup hulled hemp seeds

1 teaspoon ground cinnamon

½ teaspoon sea salt

1 pitted date (optional)

In a blender jar, combine the hemp seeds and 4 cups water, and process on high for 1 to 2 minutes. Add the cinnamon, sea salt, and date (if using) and process until smooth. Use immediately or transfer to an airtight storage container and refrigerate for 4 to 5 days.

Almond Milk

MAKES 4 CUPS

PREP TIME: 5 MINUTES, PLUS OVERNIGHT FOR SOAKING

1 cup raw almonds

1. In a small bowl, cover the almonds in water and soak overnight. The longer the almonds soak, the creamier the almond milk. Drain and rinse the almonds.
2. In a blender, combine the almonds and 4 cups water. Blend at the highest speed for 2 minutes.
3. Line a strainer with cheesecloth, and place over a bowl. Pour the almond mixture into the strainer.
4. Gather the cheesecloth around the almond meal and twist close. Squeeze and press with clean hands to extract as much almond milk as possible. Use immediately, or transfer to an airtight storage container and refrigerate for 4 to 5 days.

INGREDIENT TIP: For a sweetened version, try adding 2 pitted dates or 2 tablespoons maple syrup plus 1 tablespoon vanilla to the mixture before blending.

Carrot Cake Smoothie

DF GF NF Vegan

SERVES 2

PREP TIME: 5 MINUTES

½ frozen banana

½ cup nondairy milk (see page 76)

¼ cup steamed frozen sweet potato

¼ cup frozen carrots

1 date, pitted and soaked

2 teaspoons ground flaxseed

Pinch cinnamon

This smoothie is loaded with nutritious ingredients like carrots and flaxseed, and it's so delicious everyone in your family will love it, not just your toddler. Whip up a larger batch to feed the whole family a nutritious and quick breakfast. Working with frozen ingredients makes this vitamin-rich smoothie creamy with little effort. Steam, measure into single portions, and freeze a couple sweet potatoes to have on hand to make this quick meal.

In a blender, combine the banana, milk, sweet potato, carrots, date, flaxseed, and cinnamon. Process until smooth and serve. Transfer remainders to reusable pouches and store, refrigerated, for up to 3 days.

INGREDIENT TIP: To soak the date, cover it in very hot water and boil for 5 minutes. Remove from water before adding to the smoothie.

Berry Flax Smoothie Bowl

SERVES 2

PREP TIME: 5 MINUTES

1 cup nondairy milk (see page 76)

1 cup frozen blueberries

½ cup baby spinach

¼ avocado, pitted and peeled

2 tablespoons ground flaxseed

½ teaspoon fresh, grated ginger, or ¼ teaspoon ground ginger

You can thin this out with a little additional milk to make a drinkable smoothie or keep it as is for a smoothie bowl your toddler can enjoy with a spoon. While it's a little messy, practicing feeding themselves with a spoon is key to fine-motor development.

In a blender, combine the milk, blueberries, spinach, avocado, flaxseed, and ginger. Process until smooth. Serve in a bowl. If desired, garnish with a few fresh blueberries or sliced strawberries. Transfer any unoffered portion to reusable pouches and store, refrigerated, for up to 3 days.

SUBSTITUTION TIP: Mixed berries are a delicious substitution here. You can find frozen mixed berries in the freezer section of the grocery store.

Chocolate and Avocado Smoothie with Pepitas

SERVES 2

PREP TIME: 5 MINUTES

1 cup whole milk or nondairy milk (see page 76)

¼ cup plain whole-milk yogurt

1 tablespoon pure maple syrup

¼ avocado

1 tablespoon unsweetened cacao powder

2 tablespoons pepitas, soaked

½ cup crushed ice

You can also make these smoothies into ice pops by freezing them in ice pop molds, which makes them a great summertime snack for your toddler. They are lightly sweet and packed with nutritious vitamin-rich ingredients and fiber. Popsicles also make for a fun (albeit messy) breakfast if your toddler doesn't like smoothies.

In a blender, combine the milk, yogurt, maple syrup, avocado, cacao powder, pepitas, and ice. Process until smooth and serve. Transfer any unoffered portion to reusable pouches and store, refrigerated, for up to 3 days.

INGREDIENT TIP: To make the seeds easier to blend, soak the pepitas. Put them in a bowl of nearly boiling water and allow them to soak for 20 to 30 minutes, or boil them for 5 minutes on the stove top and drain.

Beet Berry Smoothie

SERVES 2

PREP TIME: 5 MINUTES

1 cup whole milk or non-dairy milk (see page 76)

1 cup frozen strawberries (or berries of your choice)

½ golden beet, cut into six small pieces

2 tablespoons sun butter

1 tablespoon chia seeds

Beets have a sweet, earthy flavor, and they are an excellent source of magnesium and folate. Their earthiness, when combined with berries, has just enough sweetness without being overwhelming. You can use fresh, frozen, canned, or roasted beets for this recipe.

In a blender, combine the milk, strawberries, beet, sun butter, and chia seeds. Process until smooth and serve. Transfer any remaining portion to reusable pouches and store, refrigerated, for up to 3 days.

METHOD TIP: You may need to start blending by pulsing the blender for about 10 (1-second) pulses before you allow it to run on purée. This helps chop the beets and frozen berries and distribute them throughout the smoothie.

INGREDIENT TIP: Red beets can dye clothing, so I opt for golden beets with kiddos. You could also use red beets, just make sure your toddler isn't wearing their Sunday best.

Fruit and Greens Smoothie

GF NF V

SERVES 2

PREP TIME: 5 MINUTES

1 cup baby spinach

1 cup whole milk

½ banana, frozen

½ pear, peeled, cored, and cubed

1 date, pitted and soaked

¼ cup plain whole-milk yogurt

Pinch nutmeg

Smoothies are a great way for your child to get their nutritious leafy greens, and Julian for one never says no to a smoothie! While this one calls for spinach, you can also use an equal amount of destemmed, chopped kale or chard in place of the spinach.

In a blender, combine the spinach, milk, banana, pear, date, yogurt, and nutmeg. Process until smooth and serve. Transfer any unoffered portion to reusable pouches and store, refrigerated, for up to 3 days.

INGREDIENT TIP: If using frozen spinach, reduce the amount to ½ cup. To soak the date, cover it in very hot water and boil for 5 minutes. Remove from water before adding to the smoothie.

Kiwi Chia Pudding

DF GF Vegan

SERVES 2

PREP TIME: 5 MINUTES

1 cup Almond Milk
(page 77) or other non-
dairy milk (see page 76)

¼ cup canned
coconut milk

2 tablespoons chia seeds

½ teaspoon
vanilla extract

Pinch sea salt

2 kiwis, peeled
and chopped

This chia pudding is a key to sane mornings at my house. I make a big batch (double this recipe), allow the pudding to sit overnight in the fridge, and this is what we eat as we head out the door. I like a nice, thick pudding.

1. In a bowl, stir together the almond milk, coconut milk, chia seeds, vanilla, and salt. Cover and refrigerate overnight.
2. Stir, top with the chopped kiwi, and serve.

SUBSTITUTION TIP: Any fruit works here. I like kiwi, but it's also good with berries, pears, chopped plums, or whatever is in season and available locally.

Yogurt, Fruit, and Seed Bowl

`GF` `NF` `V`

SERVES 2

PREP TIME: 5 MINUTES

1½ cups plain whole-milk yogurt

1 cup peaches, chopped

1 tablespoon honey (optional)

1 date, pitted and chopped

2 tablespoons hulled sunflower seeds (optional)

What could be easier than spooning some yogurt into a bowl and topping it with a sprinkling of seeds and chopped fruit? While this recipe calls for a single fruit (in this case, peaches), feel free to use any combination of fruits that are in season and available locally. You can make a larger batch of the yogurt, honey, date, and fruit purée if you wish and store it in the fridge for up to 5 days as a healthier version of fruit-on-the-bottom yogurt. Then just sprinkle with seeds and serve. Feel free to add other toppings as well, such as unsweetened shredded coconut, hemp hearts, or rolled oats.

1. In a blender, combine the yogurt, peaches, honey (if using), and date. Blend until smooth.
2. Spoon into two bowls. Sprinkle with the sunflower seeds (if using).

SUBSTITUTION TIP: If you've got a dairy-free toddler, you can substitute plain almond milk or coconut milk yogurt. For toddlers under 12 months, replace the honey with pure maple syrup or omit altogether.

Broccoli and Cheese Mini Frittata Muffins

**SERVES 6
(2 MUFFINS EACH)**

PREP TIME: 10 MINUTES
COOK TIME: 10 MINUTES

2 tablespoons extra-virgin olive oil, plus more for greasing

1 cup broccoli florets, broken into small pieces

½ red bell pepper, chopped

8 large eggs, beaten

⅓ cup Parmesan cheese, grated

Kosher salt (optional)

What's great about these mini frittata muffins is they freeze beautifully. Remove them from mini muffin tins and freeze them in a resealable bag. Heat in the microwave for 1 to 2 minutes (depending on your microwave's power) or serve them thawed but cold for meals on the go.

1. Preheat the oven to 375°F. Brush the cups of a mini muffin tin lightly with olive oil.
2. In a large nonstick skillet, heat the olive oil on medium high until it shimmers. Add the broccoli and bell pepper and cook for about 5 minutes, stirring occasionally, until soft. Remove from the heat, and cool for 5 minutes.
3. In a medium bowl, combine the eggs, cooled vegetable mix, and Parmesan cheese. Pour into the prepared muffin tins and bake for 10 minutes, until set.
4. Season with salt (if using).

SUBSTITUTION TIP: Leeks are a great substitute for broccoli here, if they are seasonally available.

Oat and Cranberry Breakfast Cookies

**SERVES 6 TO 8
(2 COOKIES EACH)**

PREP TIME: 10 MINUTES
COOK TIME: 20 MINUTES

2 cups rolled oats

2 very ripe
bananas, mashed

1 large egg

1 cup unsweetened
applesauce

½ teaspoon ground
cinnamon

½ teaspoon fresh
ginger, grated

½ teaspoon
vanilla extract

¼ cup dried cranberries

The beauty of cookies for breakfast is that you can freeze a large batch and thaw one or two when you're in a hurry. When your cookies are loaded with healthy ingredients like these, they also make a nutritious snack any time of day. These cookies contain no added sugar and are an excellent source of fiber and vitamins. The next time your toddler asks for a cookie, you can feel good about handing them one of these. For gluten-free cookies, be sure you purchase gluten-free oats.

1. Preheat the oven to 350°F. Line a baking sheet with parchment paper.
2. In a large bowl, combine the oats, bananas, egg, applesauce, cinnamon, ginger, vanilla, and cranberries. Stir to mix well.
3. Drop by tablespoons onto the prepared baking sheet. Bake for about 20 minutes, until the cookies are golden. Serve warm or cold.

SUBSTITUTION TIP: You can use commercially prepared unsweetened applesauce or replace with the Beet Applesauce (page 103).

Whole-Grain Waffles

NF V

SERVES 6

PREP TIME: 10 MINUTES
COOK TIME: 10 MINUTES

¼ cups melted coconut
oil, plus extra for greasing

1¾ cups whole milk
or nondairy milk (see
page 76)

2 large eggs, beaten

1 teaspoon
vanilla extract

1 tablespoon honey

¼ cup unsweetened
applesauce

1 cup whole-wheat flour

¾ cup ground flaxseed

¼ cup all-purpose flour

1 tablespoon
baking powder

Pinch kosher salt

Forget store-bought frozen waffles. Make a big batch of these, freeze them, and then reheat them in the toaster as you need them. They are quick and easy and you know exactly what's in them. For example, flaxseed is high in healthy omega-3 fatty acids. Top with fruit, nut butter, yogurt, or applesauce for a tasty meal.

1. Preheat a waffle iron and lightly brush it with coconut oil.
2. In a medium bowl, whisk together the melted coconut oil, milk, eggs, vanilla, honey, and applesauce.
3. Whisk in the whole-wheat flour, flaxseed, all-purpose flour, baking powder, and salt until smooth.
4. Fill a ¼-cup measuring cup with the batter and pour into the preheated waffle iron. Cook for about 4 minutes, until crisp and brown. Repeat with the remaining batter. Serve warm.

SUBSTITUTION TIP: For younger children (under 12 months), replace the honey with 1 tablespoon of pure maple syrup.

COOKING TIP: You can also use this as pancake batter if you don't have a waffle iron. Just use a scant ¼ cup on an oiled, nonstick grill on medium high and cook until bubbles form, about 3 minutes. Flip and cook the other side an additional 3 minutes.

Baked Oatmeal Raisin Cookie Oatmeal

NF V

SERVES 6

PREP TIME: 10 MINUTES
COOK TIME: 45 MINUTES

2 tablespoons melted coconut oil, plus extra for greasing

1½ cups unsweetened applesauce

1½ cups whole milk or nondairy milk (see page 76)

1 large egg

2 tablespoons pure maple syrup

½ teaspoon vanilla extract

1 teaspoon ground cinnamon

½ teaspoon ground nutmeg

¼ teaspoon kosher salt

1 teaspoon baking powder

3 cups rolled oats

½ cup raisins

Baked oatmeal keeps well, making it a perfect weekday breakfast. Bake up a batch on the weekend, refrigerate it, and reheat it on busy mornings for a quick and nutritious breakfast. It will keep in the fridge for up to 5 days.

1. Preheat the oven to 375°F. Grease a 9-by-9-inch square casserole with coconut oil.
2. In a bowl, whisk together the coconut oil, applesauce, milk, egg, maple syrup, vanilla, cinnamon, nutmeg, salt, and baking powder.
3. Stir in the oats and raisins.
4. Pour into the prepared baking dish. Bake for 45 minutes, until browned and set.

SUBSTITUTION TIP: For younger children (under 12 months), replace the honey with 1 tablespoon of pure maple syrup. For gluten-free, be sure you purchase gluten-free oats.

Apple Breakfast Quinoa

SERVES 4

PREP TIME: 10 MINUTES
COOK TIME: 20 MINUTES

1 tablespoon coconut oil

1 sweet-tart apple, such as a Braeburn, peeled, cored, and chopped

1 teaspoon ground cinnamon

1 cup quinoa

1½ cups water

You can make this simple breakfast quinoa with any fruit; pears are an especially tasty substitution. If desired, top with unsweetened applesauce or a tablespoon of pure maple syrup. This will refrigerate well—it will keep up to 5 days in the fridge, and you can enjoy it reheated or chilled.

1. In a large pot, heat the coconut oil on medium high until it shimmers. Add the apple and cook for about 5 minutes, stirring occasionally, until soft.
2. Add the ground cinnamon and quinoa and cook for 1 minute while stirring.
3. Add the water and bring to a boil. Reduce the heat, cover, and simmer for about 15 minutes, until the quinoa is fluffy.

SERVING TIP: You can enjoy this as is or like you would a traditional oatmeal, with milk poured over the top.

Pumpkin Overnight Oats

NF V

SERVES 2

PREP TIME: 10 MINUTES,
PLUS 1 HOUR TO CHILL

1½ cups whole milk
or nondairy milk (see
page 76)

1 cup rolled oats

⅓ cup canned
pumpkin purée

2 tablespoons sun butter

1 tablespoon pure
maple syrup

1 teaspoon ground
cinnamon

Pinch sea salt

2 tablespoons pepitas
(optional)

This quick, overnight recipe is so easy and really delicious. It's a favorite of mine because it's perfect for busy mornings, and cleanup is minimal. It's also customizable so you can eliminate any allergens by using gluten-free oats or nondairy milk.

1. In a large mason jar, combine the milk, oats, pumpkin purée, sun butter, maple syrup, cinnamon, and salt. Seal tightly and shake.
2. Refrigerate overnight.
3. Top with pepitas (if using) to serve.

SERVING TIP: If dairy isn't an issue, you can replace the sun butter with an equal amount of Greek yogurt, or if nuts aren't an issue, you can replace it with any nut butter you choose.

Banana and Egg Pancakes

SERVES 2

PREP TIME: 5 MINUTES
COOK TIME: 10 MINUTES

2 very ripe
bananas, mashed

2 large eggs, beaten

1 tablespoon whole-
wheat flour

1 tablespoon ground
flaxseed

½ teaspoon ground
cinnamon

Coconut oil, for cooking

With just a few ingredients, these truly are the world's easiest pancakes. They're also a great way to use up overripe bananas—the riper, the better. They will freeze well, and you can reheat them in the microwave.

1. In a small bowl, mix the bananas, eggs, flour, flaxseed, and cinnamon until well combined.
2. Heat a nonstick skillet on medium high. Add the coconut oil and heat until it shimmers, swirling to coat the pan.
3. Using a ¼-cup measuring cup, drop the pancake batter into the pan. Cook for about 4 minutes, until bubbles form in the top, and flip the pancakes. Cook another 2 to 3 minutes.

SERVING TIP: Top with berries, pure maple syrup, honey, nut butter, or apple-sauce, or serve with plain yogurt whisked with cinnamon and a bit of honey for dipping. With a little creativity, these can be turned into fun animal shapes using fruit and nut butter!

Chocolate Chip Oat Banana Blender Muffins

**SERVES 6 TO 8
(1 MUFFIN EACH)**

PREP TIME: 10 MINUTES
COOK TIME: 15 TO
20 MINUTES

Coconut oil, for greasing

2 cups rolled oats

3 bananas

2 large eggs

½ cup pitted dates

1 teaspoon baking soda

¼ cup chocolate chips

Blender muffins have been a game changer in our household. They are free of flour and refined sugar and are the perfect on-the-go healthy breakfast, snack, or side dish. Our whole family loves them. All you need is a blender and a muffin tin.

1. Preheat the oven to 350°F. Lightly grease a muffin tin with coconut oil.
2. In a blender, pulse the oats until a coarse powder forms. You may need to do this in batches. Add the bananas, eggs, dates, and baking soda, and pulse again. Pour into the muffin tin cups, and top with the chocolate chips.
3. Bake for 15 to 20 minutes until set and lightly browned.

MAKE-AHEAD TIP: They freeze extremely well! So make a big batch to have on hand for busy weeks.

Apple Sandwiches with Cashew Butter

SERVES 2

PREP TIME: 5 MINUTES

8 thin apple slices

2 tablespoons
cashew butter

1 teaspoon honey

Breakfast on the go doesn't get any easier than these quick apple sandwiches. Slice your apples very thin so the sandwiches are easy for toddler teeth to bite through.

1. Spread 4 of the apple slices with the cashew butter.
2. Drizzle with the honey and top with the remaining apple slices.

SUBSTITUTION TIP: To make these nut-free, substitute sun butter for the cashew butter.

Avocado Toast Toads in a Hole

SERVES 2

PREP TIME: 5 MINUTES
COOK TIME: 10 MINUTES

2 whole-grain bread slices

2 tablespoons unsalted butter

2 large eggs

¼ cup avocado, mashed

Pinch sea salt

Both toads in a hole and avocado toast make a tasty breakfast, but when you combine the two, it's even better! This breakfast is quick, easy, and nutritious. You can also make it gluten-free if you use gluten-free sandwich bread.

1. Cut a 3-inch hole in the center of each piece of bread. Use a cookie cutter if you have one to create a fun shape.
2. In a large, nonstick skillet, melt the butter on medium high until it bubbles.
3. Put the toast in the pan and carefully crack an egg into the center of each piece of toast.
4. Cook for 3 minutes, or until the whites begin to set. Flip and cook 3 minutes more.
5. Spread the avocado around the eggs on the toast.
6. Season with sea salt.

COOKING TIP: It may help to pre-crack the eggs into a custard cup. Then, carefully pour the eggs into the hole in the toast from the cup.

Egg and Spinach Cake with Feta

SERVES 12

PREP TIME: 10 MINUTES
COOK TIME: 20 MINUTES

Extra-virgin olive oil, for greasing

2 cups frozen spinach, defrosted and squeezed of excess water

12 large eggs, beaten

½ teaspoon kosher salt

1 teaspoon dried thyme

1 teaspoon garlic powder

1 cup feta cheese, crumbled

This is another good recipe to bake on the weekend, freeze, and reheat during the week. Reheat in the microwave from frozen for 1 to 2 minutes on high depending on your microwave's power. You can also reheat by wrapping them in foil and putting them in a 350°F oven for about 15 minutes or serve them cold. Freeze any extras in resealable bags to keep on hand for busy mornings.

1. Preheat the oven to 350°F. Brush a 12-cup muffin tin lightly with olive oil.
2. Evenly distribute the spinach in the bottom of the muffin cups.
3. In a small bowl, whisk together the eggs, salt, thyme, and garlic powder. Pour over the spinach in the muffin tins.
4. Sprinkle with the feta cheese.
5. Bake for 18 to 20 minutes, until set.

COOKING TIP: To squeeze water out of the spinach, put it in a colander and press it with a spatula. Alternatively, roll it in a tea towel and wring it over the sink.

Sweet Potato Hash with Scrambled Eggs

SERVES 4

PREP TIME: 10 MINUTES
COOK TIME: 15 MINUTES

2 tablespoons extra-
virgin olive oil

2 sweet potatoes, peeled
and chopped into
½-inch pieces

½ yellow onion,
finely chopped

½ teaspoon kosher salt

1 teaspoon dried thyme

8 large eggs, beaten

Hash is a tasty breakfast food, and you can use any root vegetables you'd like here in place of the sweet potatoes. Carrots, potatoes, and parsnips all work well. This keeps well in the fridge for up to 5 days. Serve it with the Homemade Ketchup (page 141) for dipping.

1. In a large, nonstick skillet, heat the olive oil on medium high until it shimmers.
2. Add the sweet potatoes, onion, salt, and thyme, and cook for about 10 minutes, stirring occasionally, until the sweet potatoes begin to brown.
3. In another nonstick skillet, add the eggs. Cook, stirring occasionally, for about 4 minutes, until the eggs are set. Serve the hash with the eggs on the side.

SUBSTITUTION TIP: You can also use squash (summer or winter) in place of the sweet potato. For summer squash like zucchini, cut cooking time to about 7 minutes before adding the eggs. For winter squash like butternut, cook as directed above.

Tofu and Veggie Scramble

SERVES 2

PREP TIME: 10 MINUTES
COOK TIME: 10 MINUTES

2 tablespoons extra-virgin olive oil

¼ yellow onion, finely chopped

½ red bell pepper, chopped

6 ounces extra-firm tofu, chopped

¼ teaspoon kosher salt

1 cup baby spinach

Tofu makes a great egg substitute for a breakfast scramble that's packed with vegan protein and lots of flavor. You can use any seasonal veggies that are available locally in this scramble.

1. In a large, nonstick skillet, heat the olive oil on medium high until it shimmers.
2. Add the onion, bell pepper, tofu, and salt. Cook for about 7 minutes, stirring occasionally, until the veggies and tofu are browned.
3. Add the spinach and cook 1 minute more, stirring until soft.

SUBSTITUTION TIP: You can replace the spinach with an equal amount of destemmed and finely chopped kale. Add the kale at the same time you add the other vegetables and cook it for the full 7 minutes.

Simple Scramble with Chicken Sausage

SERVES 4

PREP TIME: 10 MINUTES
COOK TIME: 10 MINUTES

4 ounces ground chicken

1 teaspoon dried sage

1 teaspoon garlic powder

Pinch red pepper flakes (optional)

½ teaspoon sea salt

2 tablespoons extra-virgin olive oil

6 large eggs, beaten

This recipe includes a super easy homemade chicken sausage made from ground chicken. If you don't want to make your own chicken sausage, you can buy premade chicken sausage and use it instead. If you do make your own sausage, you can make a larger batch, cook it, and store it in the freezer in single servings for use in other recipes. The entire breakfast will freeze or refrigerate well, and you can reheat it in the microwave as needed.

1. In a small bowl, mix together the chicken, sage, garlic powder, red pepper flakes (if using), and salt, mixing well.
2. In a large, nonstick skillet, heat the olive oil on medium high until it shimmers.
3. Add the chicken mixture and cook for about 5 minutes, crumbling with a spoon, until it is browned.
4. Add the eggs. Cook for about 4 minutes, stirring occasionally, until the eggs are cooked through.

COOKING TIP: Mix the sausage with clean hands to ensure the herbs and spices are evenly distributed throughout.

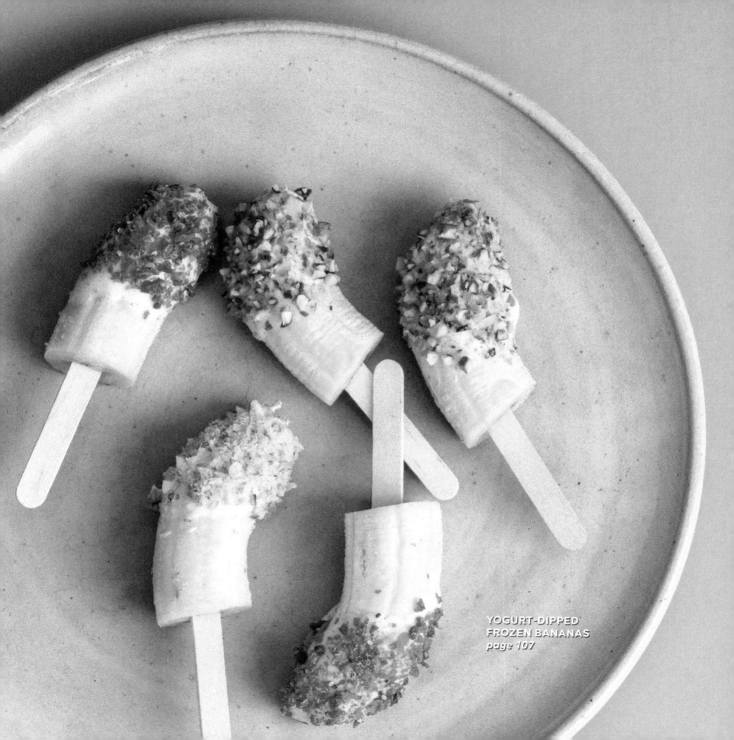

YOGURT-DIPPED
FROZEN BANANAS
page 107

6

SNACKS

Snacking is a good way to help keep your toddler's nutrition and energy levels up during the day. However, it's important you understand your toddler doesn't need to constantly be snacking. Instead, consider only having one or two snacks per day (one in the morning and one in the afternoon), and make them small so they won't disrupt meals. Along with the recipes in this chapter, fruits and vegetables also make excellent snacks.

Maple Spice Pepita Trail Mix

SERVES 4

PREP TIME: 5 MINUTES
COOK TIME: 20 MINUTES

1 cup pepitas

3 tablespoons pure
maple syrup

¼ teaspoon
ground ginger

¼ cup dried cranberries

Pinch sea salt

Pepitas, which are hulled pumpkin seeds, are a great source of fiber and protein, and they are a good source of potassium, iron, and magnesium. They're also delicious, especially when baked with lots of maple syrup and dried cranberries. This mix will keep for up to a week tightly sealed at room temperature.

1. Preheat the oven to 300°F. Line a rimmed baking sheet with parchment paper.
2. In a small bowl, mix the pepitas, maple syrup, and ginger. Spread in a single layer on the prepared baking sheet.
3. Bake for about 20 minutes, stirring once or twice, until golden.
4. Return to the bowl. Stir in the cranberries and season with the salt.

SUBSTITUTION TIP: You can also use hulled sunflower seeds in place of the pepitas, or use a mix of the two. Oat cereal (like Cheerios) also works well. You can use dried cherries, blueberries, apples, or raisins in place of the cranberries, and you can replace the syrup with an equal amount of honey.

Sweet Potato Toasts with Avocado

SERVES 4

PREP TIME: 5 MINUTES
COOK TIME: 10 MINUTES

½ sweet potato, peeled and sliced lengthwise into ¼-inch-thick slices

¼ avocado, mashed

2 teaspoons freshly squeezed lime juice

Pinch sea salt

Sweet potato toasts make a super quick snack, and they're remarkably versatile because you can customize your toppings. You can make the toasts ahead of time if you wish. Store them in a resealable bag in the fridge for up to a week and reheat in the toaster.

1. In a toaster, heat the slices of sweet potatoes for 5 to 10 minutes, until cooked through and tender. You may need to pop them back in the toaster a few times depending on your toaster settings.
2. In a small bowl, mash the avocado with the lime and salt.
3. Spread on the sweet potato toasts just before serving.

SUBSTITUTION TIP: Toppings are limited only by imagination. You can spread the veggie toasts with apple butter, Maple Butternut Butter (page 113), a thick fruit or veggie purée, tahini, nut butter, or honey.

Roasted Delicata Squash with Honey Butter

SERVES 4

PREP TIME: 5 MINUTES
COOK TIME: 20 MINUTES

1 delicata squash, halved lengthwise and cut into ¼-to ½-inch-thick slices

1 tablespoon unsalted butter, melted

1 tablespoon honey

¼ teaspoon ground cinnamon

Pinch sea salt

These squash slices are delicious warm, or you can cool them off and pack them to go. They'll keep in the fridge for up to 5 days, and they have a light, sweet flavor your toddler will love.

1. Preheat the oven to 350°F. Line a rimmed baking sheet with parchment paper.
2. In a large bowl, toss the squash with the butter, honey, cinnamon, and salt. Spread in a single layer on the prepared baking sheet.
3. Bake for 20 minutes, turning once, until tender.

SUBSTITUTION TIP: For vegan and dairy-free, replace the butter with melted coconut oil and replace the honey with pure maple syrup.

Beet Applesauce

DF GF NF Vegan

SERVES 4 TO 6

PREP TIME: 5 MINUTES
COOK TIME: 30 MINUTES

**2 beets, peeled
and chopped**

**3 sweet-tart apples, such
as Braeburn, peeled,
cored, and chopped**

**1 tablespoon freshly
squeezed lemon juice**

**½ teaspoon ground
cinnamon**

**½ teaspoon fresh
ginger, grated**

Pinch sea salt

I stumbled on this recipe experimenting in the kitchen and trying to jazz up my applesauce a bit. The beet flavor is subtly sweet and earthy and pairs well with the apples. You can put this in reusable pouches and take as an on-the-go snack. Freeze for up to 6 months or refrigerate for up to 5 days.

1. In a large pot, combine the beets and ½ cup water. Simmer for 15 minutes, uncovered, stirring occasionally.
2. Add the apples, lemon juice, cinnamon, ginger, and salt. Simmer for 10 to 15 minutes, stirring occasionally, until saucy.
3. Cool slightly and, if desired, blend with an immersion blender, in a food processor, or in a blender to make the sauce smooth.

INGREDIENT TIP: I used red beets for my applesauce because I love the color they add. However, you can use any type of beet here. If you are concerned about staining, you can use golden beets.

Carrot Fries with Citrus-Tahini Dipping Sauce

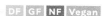

SERVES 4

PREP TIME: 10 MINUTES
COOK TIME: 20 MINUTES

3 carrots, peeled, halved crosswise, and cut into ½-inch spears

2 tablespoons extra-virgin olive oil

¼ teaspoon sea salt

¼ cup tahini

1 garlic clove, minced

3 tablespoons freshly squeezed lemon or orange juice

2 tablespoons fresh parsley, chopped

Salt

Who says fries need to be made of potatoes? Using carrots adds nutrition, and baking them makes these tasty fries a flavorful alternative to French fries with a texture that is similar. You can also use the simple and tasty Homemade Ketchup (page 141) as a dipping sauce in place of the tahini.

1. Preheat the oven to 425°F.
2. In a bowl, toss the carrots with the olive oil. Spread in a single layer on a rimmed baking sheet.
3. Bake for 10 minutes. Flip and continue cooking until crispy, about 10 minutes more.
4. Season with the salt.
5. In a small bowl, whisk together the tahini, garlic, lemon juice, parsley, and 2 tablespoons water. Taste and season with salt. Serve the fries with the dipping sauce on the side.

SUBSTITUTION TIP: Daikon radish is a great substitute for carrots here, yielding similar texture and a mild, earthy flavor.

Chewy Nut-Free Granola Bars

SERVES 8

PREP TIME: 10 MINUTES
COOK TIME: 15 MINUTES

2 cups rolled oats

⅔ cup ground flaxseed

1 cup dried
dates, chopped

1 cup dried
apples, chopped

½ cup extra-virgin
olive oil

½ cup pure maple syrup

¼ cup raw honey

Using gluten-free oats makes these bars allergen-free. They're also quick to mix and super easy to make, and they keep well at room temperature for up to a week. They're perfect snacks for busy parents, toddlers, and older siblings, and they're also great for lunchboxes or picnics.

1. Preheat the oven to 350°F. Line a 9-by-13-inch baking pan with parchment paper.
2. In a large bowl, mix together the oats, flaxseed, dates, apples, olive oil, maple syrup, and honey. Press into the prepared baking pan.
3. Bake for 15 minutes, until golden.
4. Cut into squares to serve.

SUBSTITUTION TIP: To make this vegan (or for babies under 12 months old), replace the honey with 2 tablespoons pure maple syrup.

Peach Toast with Maple Tahini

SERVES 1

PREP TIME: 10 MINUTES
COOK TIME: 5 MINUTES

1 whole-grain bread slice,
toasted and halved

½ peach, thinly sliced

2 tablespoons tahini

1 tablespoon pure
maple syrup

Whole-grain toast with toppings is a great snack for toddlers. In this case, I used thinly sliced peaches, but you can use other soft fruits that are in season. This checks all the snack boxes because the protein and fats come from the tahini and fiber comes from the peach and bread.

1. Arrange the toast on a plate. Put the peach slices on top of the toast.
2. In a small bowl, whisk together the tahini and syrup. Drizzle over the peaches.

SUBSTITUTION TIP: You can also drizzle with a honey-yogurt sauce in place of the tahini and maple syrup. In a small bowl, whisk together ¼ cup plain yogurt with 1 tablespoon of honey and drizzle it over the fruit.

Pumpkin Muffin Minis

GF NF V

SERVES 12

PREP TIME: 10 MINUTES
COOK TIME: 15 MINUTES

Coconut oil, melted, for greasing

2 cups gluten-free rolled oats

2 tablespoons hemp hearts

½ teaspoon ground cinnamon

¼ teaspoon ground nutmeg

Pinch sea salt

Pinch baking powder

1 cup pumpkin purée

1 large egg, beaten

1 cup whole milk or non-dairy milk (see page 76)

¼ cup pure maple syrup

½ teaspoon vanilla extract

These mini muffins take a few minutes to bake, but it's passive time where you can be doing something else. They keep well, up to 1 week tightly sealed, and they freeze really well, up to 6 months. So they are perfect for making on a weekend and grabbing one when your toddler needs a quick, nutritious snack. I know Julian sure loves when I pull these out of the freezer!

1. Preheat the oven to 350°F. Brush the muffin tins lightly with melted coconut oil.
2. In a large bowl, whisk together the oats, hemp hearts, cinnamon, nutmeg, salt, and baking powder.
3. In another bowl, whisk together the pumpkin, egg, milk, maple syrup, and vanilla.
4. Add the wet ingredients to the dry, mixing until just combined.
5. Spoon into the prepared muffin tins. Bake for 12 to 15 minutes, until a toothpick inserted in the center comes out clean.

INGREDIENT TIP: You can find hemp hearts online or at your local health food store. If you can't find them, substitute an equal amount of chia or flaxseed.

Yogurt-Dipped Frozen Bananas

SERVES 4

PREP TIME: 10 MINUTES, PLUS 3 TO 6 HOURS FREEZING TIME

2 bananas, halved lengthwise

1 cup plain whole-milk yogurt

2 tablespoons pure maple syrup

½ teaspoon ground cinnamon

These frozen bananas are so much fun for toddlers to decorate. You can have your little one roll them in coconut, goji berries, or crushed nuts, or use raisins, mini chocolate chips, or other small dried fruits to decorate them. I made them into ghosts for Halloween, using the raisins as eyes, and Julian just loved them! Use either ice pop sticks or wooden skewers for these fun treats. If you use wooden skewers, be sure to cut the pointy tip off before assembling.

1. Line a baking sheet with parchment paper.
2. Insert ice pop sticks or skewers into the bananas along the cut edge.
3. In a medium bowl, whisk together the yogurt, maple syrup, and cinnamon.
4. Dip the bananas in the yogurt, coating them. Arrange on the prepared baking sheet.
5. Decorate as desired.
6. Freeze for 3 to 6 hours or until the yogurt is set.

INGREDIENT TIP: To make this dairy-free and vegan, you can use a plain coconut or almond milk yogurt.

Pumpkin Energy Balls

DF GF NF V

SERVES 10 TO 12

PREP TIME: 10 MINUTES

1½ cups gluten-free rolled oats

½ cup sun butter

½ cup pumpkin purée

¼ cup ground flaxseed

¼ cup honey

½ teaspoon pumpkin pie spice

Pinch sea salt

These no-bake pumpkin balls are tasty, and they freeze well so they're perfect on-the-go snacks your toddler (and probably everyone else in your family) will enjoy. I also find with energy bites that you can really add anything to them. Check what's in your pantry—these would be excellent with shredded coconut, dried fruit, or cacao powder added in. Use gluten-free oats to keep them gluten- and allergen-free.

1. Line a baking sheet with parchment paper.
2. In a medium bowl, combine the oats, sun butter, pumpkin purée, flaxseed, honey, pumpkin pie spice, and salt, mixing well.
3. Form the mixture into 1-tablespoon balls and place on the prepared tray. Serve immediately, or transfer to an airtight container and store, refrigerated, for up to 1 week.

SUBSTITUTION TIP: For vegan, you can replace the honey with 3 tablespoons of pure maple syrup. You may need to add up to ¼ cup more of the oats to adjust the texture of the balls.

Avocado Fries

SERVES 4

PREP TIME: 10 MINUTES
COOK TIME: 15 MINUTES

1 avocado, cut into lengthwise spears

Juice of ¼ lime

¼ cup almond flour

½ teaspoon sea salt

1 egg, beaten

The soft texture of these baked avocado bites makes them easy for little ones to eat, and they enjoy the crispy coating. You can serve with a dip, such as ranch dressing or another favorite to make this a fun toddler snack.

1. Preheat the oven to 400°F. Line a baking sheet with parchment paper.
2. Sprinkle lime juice over the avocado pieces.
3. In a small bowl, combine the almond flour and sea salt.
4. In a small bowl, whisk the egg.
5. Dip the avocado pieces into the egg and then into the almond flour mixture.
6. Arrange on the prepared baking sheet. Bake for 15 minutes, or until crisp.

INGREDIENT TIP: To prevent browning, you can rub the cut half of a lime directly on the avocado before you sprinkle them with the lime juice.

Banana Sushi Bites

SERVES 2

PREP TIME: 10 MINUTES

2 tablespoons cashew or almond butter

1 whole-wheat tortilla

1 banana, peeled

Pinch ground cinnamon, for garnish

Sushi for toddlers? Sure, if you're making it from banana and tortillas. Your toddler will love these fun shapes, and it's a great way to offer foods in a different format. If you want, serve with a simple honey and yogurt sauce for dipping.

1. Spread the cashew butter on the tortilla.
2. Place the banana on the nut butter and roll, using a bit more nut butter to glue the edges shut.
3. Cut into 1½-inch-thick slices. Garnish with cinnamon.

SUBSTITUTION TIP: To make these nut-free, replace the cashew or almond butter with sun butter or tahini.

Zucchini Dip with Veggies

SERVES 4

PREP TIME: 10 MINUTES

1 medium zucchini, roughly chopped

1 tablespoon freshly squeezed lemon juice

1 garlic clove, minced

2 tablespoons tahini

2 tablespoons extra-virgin olive oil

1 tablespoon fresh parsley, chopped

Pinch sea salt

Pinch paprika

1 cucumber, peeled and cut into sticks

Zucchini makes a great base for a dip, and it doesn't require any cooking or roasting. Mix it up in the blender or food processor with some spices and a touch of tahini, and it's a great-tasting veggie-based dip your toddler can use for dipping other vegetables, giving them a double dose of raw nutrient-packed vegetables.

1. In a blender or food processor jar, combine the zucchini, lemon juice, garlic, tahini, olive oil, parsley, salt, and paprika. Process until smooth.
2. Serve with the cucumber sticks for dipping.

SUBSTITUTION TIP: You can change up the flavors here, as well. Replace the lemon juice with lime juice, replace the tahini with ¼ avocado, and replace the parsley with cilantro for a dip with Latin American flare.

Avocado Dipping Sauce

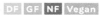

MAKES ABOUT ¼ CUP

PREP TIME: 10 MINUTES

½ avocado

1 teaspoon freshly
squeezed lime juice

½ teaspoon minced garlic

This simple sauce is going to become a go-to favorite after you realize how easy it is to transform these three ingredients into something so tasty. Use this for dipping the Cauliflower Tots (page 62), Celery Root and Sweet Potato Cakes (page 61), or just some cut vegetables for a delicious snack perfect for any time of day.

1. In a small bowl, combine the avocado, lime juice, and garlic. Using a fork, mash the avocado, mixing it together with the lime juice and garlic.

2. Add a little water, 1 teaspoon at a time, if necessary, to adjust the consistency. Serve with vegetables for dipping. Store remaining dipping sauce in the refrigerator.

INGREDIENT TIP: To prevent the avocado dip from browning during storage, cover with plastic wrap, sealing it tightly around the edges and pressing out as much air as possible.

Maple Butternut Butter

DF GF **NF** Vegan

SERVES 6

PREP TIME: 5 MINUTES
COOK TIME: 25 MINUTES

1 butternut squash, rind removed and cut into ½-inch cubes

1 tablespoon extra-virgin olive oil

¼ cup pure maple syrup

½ teaspoon ground cinnamon

2 tablespoons freshly squeezed orange juice

Pinch salt

This is a different take on apple butter. Roasting the squash gives it a rich, sweet earthiness that mixes well with maple flavors. Serve it on whole-grain toast, as a topping for the Sweet Potato Toasts with Avocado (page 101), or use it as a dip for fruit slices. This will keep in the fridge for up to 5 days or in the freezer for up to 6 months.

1. Preheat the oven to 425°F.
2. In a mixing bowl, toss the squash with the olive oil. Spread in a single layer on a rimmed baking sheet.
3. Bake for 20 to 25 minutes, until soft.
4. Transfer the squash to the blender or food processor along with the maple syrup, cinnamon, orange juice, and salt. Blend until smooth.

SUBSTITUTION TIP: An equal amount of any winter squash works well here, as do carrots (use about 4) or sweet potatoes (use 2).

Veggie Purée Pouches

DF GF NF Vegan

SERVES 4

PREP TIME: 5 MINUTES
COOK TIME: 10 MINUTES

1 cup diced vegetables (such as carrots, peas, or turnips)

½ cup diced, peeled fruit (such as apples or pears)

¼ cup liquid (such as unsalted vegetable broth, water, or milk)

½ teaspoon dried herbs or spices

Pinch salt

Remember all the purées you made when your toddler was a baby? When you put them in reusable pouches, they make excellent snacks while you are out and about. You can get crafty with your fruit and veggie combinations and add any herbs or spices that appeal to you. You can also heat the purées, thin them slightly, and serve them in a bowl as soup or as a soup base with small vegetables cut up in them. There is something magical about pouches—even 4- and 5-year-olds will ask for them!

1. Fill a large saucepan with 1 inch of water and insert a steamer basket. Bring the water to a boil.
2. Add the vegetables and fruit to the steamer basket and steam for 10 minutes, until soft.
3. Transfer to a blender or food processor. Add the liquid, a couple tablespoons at a time, along with the herbs and salt. Purée until smooth, adjusting the thickness by adding more liquid as needed.

INGREDIENT TIP: Try any of the following for a delicious combination: 1 cup peas, ½ cup pears, water, and nutmeg; 1 cup carrots, ½ cup apples, vegetable broth, and cinnamon; 1 cup spinach, ½ cup peaches, vegetable broth or water, and dried thyme.

Kale Chips

DF GF **NF** **Vegan**

SERVES 4 TO 6

PREP TIME: 5 MINUTES
COOK TIME: 15 MINUTES

1 kale bunch, stemmed and torn into smaller pieces

1 tablespoon extra-virgin olive oil

½ teaspoon sea salt

Getting your toddler involved in the cooking process not only serves as great together time, but it also gives them a stake in what you're cooking, making them more likely to give it a try. Kale chips are one of my son's favorite things to make with me. He rips the kale into small pieces and helps stir in seasonings.

1. Preheat the oven to 350°F. Line two rimmed baking sheets with parchment paper.
2. In a mixing bowl, toss the kale with the olive oil, and spread it in a single layer on the prepared baking sheets.
3. Bake for 10 to 15 minutes, until the edges brown.
4. Sprinkle with the salt while warm.

SUBSTITUTION TIP: Add flavor to the chips by combining ¼ teaspoon of garlic or onion powder along with the salt. You can also replace the olive oil with toasted sesame oil.

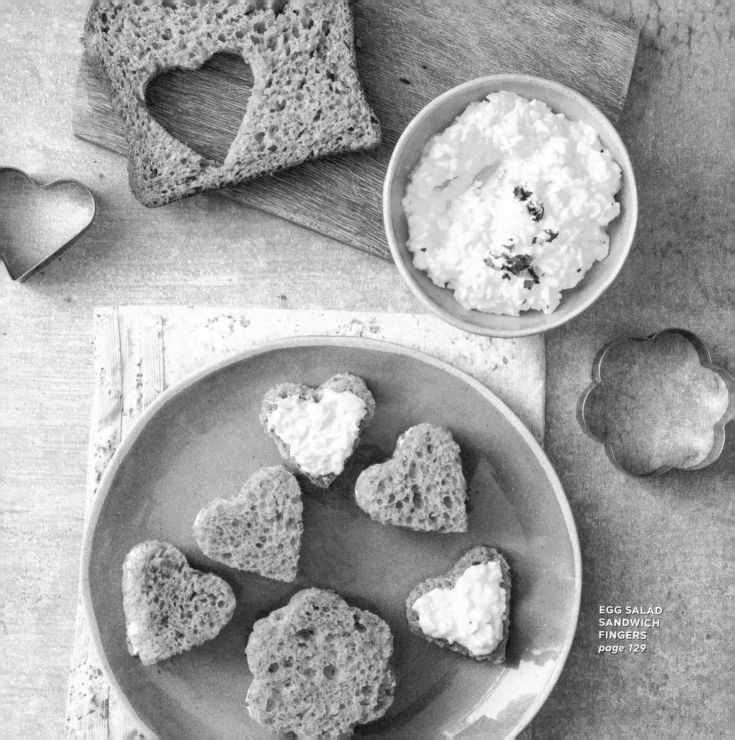

EGG SALAD
SANDWICH
FINGERS
page 129

7

LUNCH

Lunch to me is the hardest meal of the day. Most of us treat lunch as more fuel than food and typically eat it while working or on the go. Lunch, however, is really important as it helps your toddler recover from a busy morning and fuel their body before their afternoon nap. The key is to create easy, quick meals like the Tuna Avocado Wraps (page 128) or Egg Salad Sandwich Fingers (page 129) that provide needed fuel. Working parents need lunches that pack easily for their toddlers, and many of these fit the bill. You can even send a thermos of hot soup with your little one for a quick and nutritious lunch that's easy for care providers to serve. Lunch does not need to be fancy and we provide a bunch of easy recipes as well as ideas for utilizing leftovers (a constant in my home).

Quinoa with Spinach

DF GF NF Vegan

SERVES 4

PREP TIME: 10 MINUTES
COOK TIME: 20 MINUTES

1 cup unsalted vegetable broth

½ cup quinoa

2 tablespoons extra-virgin olive oil

¼ onion, finely chopped

1 cup baby spinach, finely chopped

1 garlic clove, minced

Juice of 1 lemon

2 tablespoons fresh parsley, chopped

½ teaspoon kosher salt

This quinoa and spinach mixture is good hot or cold, so it's an equally delicious lunch or a great side for family dinner. To save time, you can cook the quinoa ahead and keep it in single-serving containers in the fridge to use as needed. This will keep well in the freezer for up to 6 months.

1. In a small saucepan, bring the vegetable broth to a boil.
2. Add the quinoa. Reduce the heat to simmer and cook for about 15 minutes, covered, stirring occasionally.
3. Turn off the heat and allow the quinoa to sit, covered, for 5 minutes more. Fluff with a fork.
4. In a large nonstick skillet, heat the olive oil on medium high until it shimmers.
5. Add the onion and cook for about 5 minutes, stirring occasionally, until soft.
6. Add the spinach and cook 1 minute more. Add the garlic and cook, stirring, for 30 seconds.
7. Add the lemon juice and quinoa. Stir to combine ingredients.
8. Remove from the heat and stir in the parsley. Season with the salt.

INGREDIENT TIP: Quinoa needs to be rinsed to remove a soapy residue called saponin, which imparts bitter flavors. Put the quinoa in a fine mesh strainer and rinse for 1 or 2 minutes under cool water, using your fingers to gently rub the quinoa to remove the saponin.

Pasta Salad with Kale Pesto

SERVES 2

PREP TIME: 10 MINUTES
COOK TIME: 10 MINUTES

2 cups cooked whole-grain rotini pasta, cooled

¼ cup black olives, chopped

1 carrot, peeled and grated

2 scallions, both white and green parts, thinly sliced

2 tablespoons extra-virgin olive oil

¼ cup kale, stemmed and chopped

1 garlic clove, minced

¼ cup walnuts

2 tablespoons Parmesan cheese, grated

2 tablespoons freshly squeezed lemon juice

This cold pasta salad is tasty and makes a great lunch or side dish. While this recipe is vegetarian, you could add some flaked salmon, chopped chicken, or canned tuna if you'd like to add protein to the dish. Store any unoffered pasta salad separately from the kale pesto and mix just before serving.

1. In a bowl, combine the pasta, olives, carrot, and scallions.
2. In a blender or food processor, combine the olive oil, kale, garlic, walnuts, Parmesan cheese, and lemon juice. Pulse for 10 to 20 (1-second) pulses, until well chopped and combined.
3. Toss the pesto with the salad and serve.

SUBSTITUTION TIP: To make this dairy-free, omit the Parmesan cheese and replace with 2 tablespoons of nutritional yeast or vegan grated cheese. To make it nut-free, replace the walnuts with pepitas or hulled sunflower seeds.

Mexican Rice Salad

SERVES 4

PREP TIME: 10 MINUTES

2 cups cooked brown rice, cold

½ red bell pepper, diced

½ cup frozen corn, cooked

½ cup canned black beans, drained

2 scallions, both white and green parts, very thinly sliced

¼ avocado, pitted and finely chopped

3 tablespoons extra-virgin olive oil

Juice of 2 limes

¼ cup fresh cilantro, chopped

½ teaspoon sea salt

This colorful salad is easy. You can make brown rice ahead of time and freeze it in ½-cup portions in the freezer for up to 6 months.

1. In a bowl, combine the rice, bell pepper, corn, black beans, scallions, and avocado.
2. In a small bowl, whisk together the olive oil, lime juice, cilantro, and salt.
3. Toss the vinaigrette with the rice.

SUBSTITUTION TIP: Add ½ cup of cooked baby shrimp or ½ cup of finely diced chicken for a protein boost.

Salmon and Avocado Salad

SERVES 2

PREP TIME: 10 MINUTES

2 tablespoons fresh tarragon, chopped

Juice of ½ orange

¼ avocado, pitted and peeled

1 teaspoon Dijon mustard

1 tablespoon extra-virgin olive oil

¼ teaspoon sea salt

¾ cup cooked flaked salmon or canned salmon

Serve this salad by itself or put it in between 2 slices of whole-grain bread to make a tasty sandwich. It will keep in the fridge for up to 3 days, but it doesn't freeze well. You can replace the salmon with chopped hard-boiled eggs to make it vegetarian, or use cooked baby shrimp.

1. In a blender or food processor, combine the tarragon, orange juice, avocado, mustard, olive oil, and salt. Process until smooth.
2. In a mixing bowl, toss the dressing with the salmon.

SUBSTITUTION TIP: For a little added crunch and flavor, you can add 2 tablespoons of finely diced fennel bulb, celery, or red bell pepper.

Herbed Chicken Salad

GF NF

SERVES 2

PREP TIME: 10 MINUTES, PLUS 1 HOUR TO CHILL

1 cup cooked chicken meat, finely chopped or shredded

1 tablespoon fresh parsley, chopped

1 tablespoon fresh dill, chopped

1 tablespoon fresh chives, chopped

¼ cup plain Greek whole-milk yogurt

2 tablespoons freshly squeezed lemon juice

1 teaspoon Dijon mustard

¼ teaspoon sea salt

If you have leftover chicken, this is a great use for it. Likewise, you can use rotisserie chicken from the grocery store, or you can steam or roast chicken and cut it into small pieces. This doesn't freeze well, but it will keep in the fridge for up to 3 days. Serve it by itself or in a sandwich.

1. In a medium bowl, combine the chicken, parsley, dill, and chives.
2. In a small bowl, whisk together the yogurt, lemon juice, mustard, and salt.
3. Toss with the chicken. Chill for an hour and serve.

SUBSTITUTION TIP: To make this vegan, replace the chicken meat with chopped tofu. You can also add ¼ cup of peas for color and texture.

Tomato Soup with Grilled Cheese Croutons

SERVES 4

PREP TIME: 10 MINUTES
COOK TIME: 20 MINUTES

1 tablespoon extra-virgin olive oil

½ onion, finely chopped

2 tablespoons tomato paste

1 garlic clove, minced

1 (14-ounce) can crushed tomatoes

2 cups unsalted vegetable broth

½ teaspoon kosher salt

1 whole-grain sandwich bread slice, halved

2 teaspoons unsalted butter, softened

3 tablespoons Cheddar cheese, grated

Tomato soup and grilled cheese are perennial childhood favorites. This version replaces a full sandwich with mini grilled cheese croutons, which is a fun twist on the original. You can use gluten-free sandwich bread to make this gluten-free, or use nondairy cheese to make it dairy-free.

1. In a medium saucepan, heat the olive oil on medium high until it shimmers.

2. Add the onion and cook for about 5 minutes, stirring regularly, until soft.

3. Add the tomato paste and cook for 5 minutes, stirring constantly.

4. Add the garlic and cook, stirring constantly, for 30 seconds.

5. Add the crushed tomatoes and vegetable broth. Bring to a simmer and cook for about 5 minutes, stirring occasionally.

6. In a blender or food processor or using an immersion blender, purée until smooth. Season with the salt.

7. Preheat a nonstick pan on medium high. Spread the butter on one side of the sandwich bread. Place a half slice, butter-side down, into the pan. Sprinkle the cheese on top of the bread and top with the second slice of bread, butter-side up. Cook, pressing with a spatula or press, for about 3 minutes, until crisp. Flip and brown the other side, pressing, 2 to 3 minutes more.

8. Cut the sandwich into small squares and float on top of the soup.

METHOD TIP: When puréeing a hot liquid in a blender or food processor, allow the chute to remain open at the top to allow steam to escape. Fold a towel two or three times and place over the lid to protect your hand from hot steam and liquid, and then press gently on the towel to hold the lid in place. Hot steam in a blender that is not vented can force the lid off and cause a mess or burns.

Lentil and Sweet Potato Soup

SERVES 4

PREP TIME: 10 MINUTES
COOK TIME: 20 MINUTES

2 tablespoons extra-virgin olive oil

1 leek, washed and finely chopped

3 cups unsalted vegetable broth

½ sweet potato, peeled and cut into ½-inch pieces

½ teaspoon dried thyme

1 (14-ounce) can of lentils, drained

½ teaspoon sea salt

This hearty vegetarian soup keeps very well. Freeze it in single-serving sizes and reheat on the stove top or in the microwave whenever you need lunch on the go. In a double batch, it also makes an excellent family supper with leftovers.

1. In a large saucepan, heat the olive oil on medium high until it shimmers.
2. Add the leek and cook for about 4 minutes, stirring occasionally, until softened.
3. Add the vegetable broth, sweet potato, and thyme. Bring to a simmer and cook for 10 to 15 minutes, until the sweet potato is tender.
4. In a blender or food processor or using an immersion blender, purée the soup until smooth. Return to the pan and return to medium-high heat.
5. Add the lentils. Cook, stirring, 3 to 4 minutes more, until the lentils are heated through. Thin with additional broth or water, if needed. Season with salt.

INGREDIENT TIP: To clean the leeks, chop and then submerge into a bowl of cold water. Swish the leeks around and allow the dirt to settle to the bottom. Pour off the water, add more, and repeat the rinsing and swishing until no dirt settles at the bottom of the bowl.

White Bean and Kale Soup

DF GF **NF**

SERVES 6

PREP TIME: 10 MINUTES
COOK TIME: 20 MINUTES

2 tablespoons extra-virgin olive oil

6 ounces bulk sweet Italian sausage

½ onion, finely chopped

½ red bell pepper, finely chopped

1 cup kale, stemmed and finely chopped

1 garlic clove, minced

5 cups unsalted vegetable broth

1 cup canned white beans, drained

1 teaspoon Italian seasoning

½ teaspoon sea salt

This is another soup that freezes very well, so it's perfect for making a large batch and freezing in 1-cup servings to reheat when you need something fast. It's also easy to make vegetarian and vegan—simply omit the sausage.

1. In a large saucepan, heat the olive oil on medium high until it shimmers.
2. Add the sausage and cook for about 5 minutes, crumbling, until it browns.
3. Add the onion, bell pepper, and kale and cook for about 5 minutes, until the vegetables soften.
4. Add the garlic and cook, stirring constantly, for 30 seconds.
5. Add the vegetable broth, white beans, and Italian seasoning. Cook, stirring occasionally, for 5 minutes. Season with the salt.

SUBSTITUTION TIP: Any small beans work well in this soup. Try canned navy or pinto beans or even lentils.

Vegetable, Tofu, and Greens Soup

DF GF NF Vegan

SERVES 4

PREP TIME: 10 MINUTES
COOK TIME: 20 MINUTES

2 tablespoons extra-virgin olive oil

½ onion, finely chopped

1 carrot, peeled and finely chopped

4 ounces tofu, finely chopped

1 cup kale, stemmed and finely chopped

1 cup baby spinach, finely chopped

1 garlic clove, minced

4 cups unsalted vegetable broth

Juice of 1 lemon

½ teaspoon sea salt

This vegan soup has a delicious, citrusy flavor that complements the greens nicely. It freezes well, and it makes a great lunch for your toddler or, in larger batches, a nice vegetarian soup dinner for your entire family.

1. In a large saucepan, heat the olive oil on medium high until it shimmers.
2. Add the onion, carrot, tofu, kale, and spinach and cook for about 5 minutes, stirring occasionally, until the veggies are soft.
3. Add the garlic and cook, stirring constantly, for 30 seconds.
4. Add the vegetable broth and bring to a simmer. Cook, stirring occasionally, for 5 minutes more.
5. Remove from the heat and stir in the lemon juice. Season with salt.

SUBSTITUTION TIP: You can use any greens in this soup. Swiss chard, beet greens, mustard greens, purslane, and collard greens will all work well here depending on what's locally and seasonally available.

Sun Butter and Banana Wraps

SERVES 2

PREP TIME: 10 MINUTES

½ banana, mashed

1 tablespoon sun butter

1 teaspoon pure
maple syrup

¼ teaspoon ground
cinnamon

1 whole-grain tortilla

Wrap sandwiches are great for toddlers who need to pack a lunch because they travel and store well. Slice the wraps into thin slices and pack them in a ziptop bag or bento box along with cut fruit for a great traveling toddler lunch.

1. In a small bowl, mash together the banana, sun butter, maple syrup, and cinnamon.
2. Spread on the tortilla. Roll, using a bit of the mixture to "glue" the tortilla shut. Cut into thin slices.

SUBSTITUTION TIP: Substitute any nut butter for the sun butter, or replace the banana with ¼ avocado for an interesting twist on this wrap. To make this gluten-free, substitute a gluten-free tortilla or wrap, or cut the crust off of gluten-free bread, put it between two pieces of parchment, and roll it out to about ¼-inch thickness and use that as a wrap.

Black Bean Wraps

SERVES 2

PREP TIME: 10 MINUTES

¼ avocado, chopped

Juice of 1 lime

¼ cup canned black beans, drained

2 tablespoons plain Greek whole-milk yogurt

1 tablespoon salsa

Pinch cumin

Pinch salt

1 whole-grain tortilla

This is another wrap that travels well. Tossing the avocado pieces with lime juice helps keep them from browning for a few hours. However, because of avocado's propensity to brown, this won't keep very well overnight, so it's best to make it on the same day your toddler will consume it.

1. In a small bowl, toss the avocado and lime juice.
2. In another small bowl, mash the black beans with the yogurt, salsa, cumin, and salt.
3. Spread the black bean mixture on the tortilla. Top with the avocado and roll, using a bit of the black beans to "glue" the edges of the wrap shut.
4. Cut into thin slices and serve.

SUBSTITUTION TIP: To make this dairy-free, omit the Greek yogurt and replace it with another tablespoon of salsa or a nondairy plain yogurt.

Tuna Avocado Wraps

SERVES 2

PREP TIME: 10 MINUTES

⅛ avocado, mashed

Juice of ½ lemon

2 teaspoons mayonnaise

1 teaspoon fresh dill, chopped

1 (5-ounce) can water-packed tuna

Pinch salt (optional)

1 whole-grain tortilla

Tuna salad is held together here with an avocado mayonnaise that adds flavor and nutritional value. You can make this gluten-free by using a gluten-free wrap or turning it into a sandwich with gluten-free sandwich bread. Store the tuna and bread separately if making ahead and assemble just before serving.

1. In a small bowl, whisk together the mashed avocado, lemon juice, mayonnaise, and dill.
2. Fold in the tuna and season with the salt (if using).
3. Spread on a whole-grain tortilla and roll. Cut into slices.

SUBSTITUTION TIP: Some toddlers are allergic to fish, some to shellfish, and some to both. If your toddler is allergic to fish, replace the tuna with baby shrimp. If your toddler is allergic to both shellfish and fish, you can replace the tuna with shredded cooked chicken, chopped hardboiled eggs, or chopped tofu.

Egg Salad Sandwich Fingers

SERVES 2

PREP TIME: 10 MINUTES

2 tablespoons
mayonnaise

½ teaspoon
Dijon mustard

2 hardboiled
eggs, chopped

1 scallion, both white
and green parts,
finely chopped

1 tablespoon fresh
parsley, chopped

2 whole-grain
sandwich bread slices,
crusts removed

Egg salad is another easy make-ahead food. Store the egg salad refrigerated for up to 3 days and assemble the sandwiches before serving or packing in a lunch. For older toddlers, you can make these into cute little sandwiches by cutting in a cookie cutter shape versus cutting them into "finger" shapes. Make this vegan by replacing the eggs with chopped tofu and ensuring you use a vegan whole-grain bread and a vegan mayo. If dairy is not a problem, you can substitute the mayonnaise with plain Greek yogurt.

1. In a small bowl, whisk together the mayonnaise and mustard.
2. Stir in the eggs, scallion, and parsley, mixing until just blended.
3. Spread the salad on one piece of the bread and top with the other.
4. Cut the sandwich crosswise into 6 "fingers" or use cookie cutters and serve.

INGREDIENT TIP: To hard boil eggs, use eggs that are about a week old because eggs that are less fresh peel better. To make them, put the eggs in a single layer in the bottom of a large saucepan and cover them with water that is at least an inch over the top of the eggs. Put the pot on the burner on high heat and bring it to a boil. Turn off the heat, cover the pot, and allow the eggs to sit for 14 minutes. Then, shock the eggs in ice water to stop the cooking. Peel under running cold water.

Turkey, Carrot, and Cream Cheese "Sushi" Rolls

`GF` `NF`

SERVES 2

PREP TIME: 10 MINUTES

2 tablespoons cream cheese, softened

½ teaspoon Dijon mustard

1 teaspoon fresh chives, chopped

3 deli turkey slices

1 carrot, peeled and grated

These simple rolls pack well, and they're fun to eat for little ones. Your toddler can even help you assemble them because they're super easy to roll and slice. These are also a great party treat because they're perfect for little fingers.

1. In a small bowl, mix the cream cheese, mustard, and chives.
2. Spread each turkey slice with the cream cheese mixture. Sprinkle with the grated carrots.
3. Roll the turkey pieces up, using a bit of the cream cheese mixture to "glue" the edges of the turkey together. Cut into slices.

SUBSTITUTION TIP: Any thinly sliced deli meat works well in these rolls. Opt for low-sodium deli meats if you can find them to keep salt levels under control.

Grilled Peanut Butter and Pear Sandwiches

SERVES 2

PREP TIME: 10 MINUTES
COOK TIME: 7 MINUTES

1 tablespoon butter, softened, divided

2 tablespoons peanut butter

2 whole-grain bread slices

2 pears, peeled, cored, and thinly sliced

¼ cup plain Greek whole-milk yogurt

2 teaspoons honey

¼ teaspoon fresh ginger, grated

These sandwiches are easy to customize, and your toddler will love the gooey nut butter and mild sweetness of the pear. For younger toddlers, cut the sandwiches into thin fingers. For older toddlers, you can use a cookie cutter to make the sandwiches a fun shape.

1. Preheat a nonstick skillet on medium high. Melt half the butter in the pan.
2. Spread the peanut butter on one side of a piece of bread and place the bare side into the melted butter in the pan. Arrange the pear slices on the bread. Spread the remaining ½ tablespoon butter on the other piece of bread and place it on the sandwich, butter-side up. Press with a spatula or use a press and cook for about 3 minutes, until golden brown. Flip the sandwich and grill, pressing, for about 3 minutes more, until golden.
3. Meanwhile, in a small bowl, whisk together the yogurt, honey, and ginger.
4. Cut the sandwich crosswise into 6 "fingers" and serve with the yogurt as a dipping sauce.

SUBSTITUTION TIP: To make this vegan and dairy-free, omit the butter and replace it with melted coconut oil and eliminate the yogurt dipping sauce. To make them nut-free, replace the peanut butter with sun butter. To make them gluten-free, use gluten-free sandwich bread.

Make-Ahead Meatloaf Muffins

NF

SERVES 6

PREP TIME: 10 MINUTES
COOK TIME: 30 MINUTES

Extra-virgin olive oil, for greasing

½ cup whole milk or non-dairy milk (see page 76)

½ cup whole-grain bread crumbs

1 pound ground beef

1 large egg, beaten

1 tablespoon Dijon mustard

1 carrot, peeled and grated

½ onion, grated

1 teaspoon dried thyme

½ teaspoon kosher salt

½ teaspoon garlic powder

The trick to keeping these mini meatloaves moist is something called a panade, which is simply mixing bread crumbs (you can use gluten-free if desired) with milk (you can use a nondairy milk if desired). While these meatloaves take a while to cook, they are a great weekend project for make-ahead meals (you can serve them cold or hot) because they keep well in the fridge or freezer.

1. Preheat the oven to 350°F. Brush a 6-muffin tin with a small amount of olive oil.
2. In a small bowl, mix the milk and bread crumbs. Allow to sit for 5 minutes.
3. In a large bowl, combine the bread crumb mixture with the ground beef, egg, mustard, carrot, onion, thyme, salt, and garlic powder.
4. Use your hands to mix well without overworking. Divide evenly among the muffin cups.
5. Bake for 25 to 30 minutes, until the internal temperature is 165°F.

SUBSTITUTION TIP: Some people prefer a mixture of meats to make the texture of their meatloaves more refined. A standard combination is 8 ounces of ground beef, 4 ounces of ground pork, and 4 ounces of ground veal. You can also make this into a loaf pan and slice it. To cook it in a loaf pan, it will take 60 to 65 minutes.

Fish Sticks with Yogurt Tartar Sauce

SERVES 8

PREP TIME: 10 MINUTES
COOK TIME: 15 MINUTES

2 large eggs, beaten

1 teaspoon
Dijon mustard

Juice of ½ lemon

2 cups bread crumbs

1 teaspoon dried thyme

1 teaspoon dried dill

1 teaspoon onion powder

½ teaspoon salt

1 pound cod, pin bones
and skin removed and
cut into strips

½ cup plain Greek whole-
milk yogurt

1 dill pickle, finely minced

½ teaspoon lemon zest

½ teaspoon fresh
tarragon, chopped

I like to double or even triple this recipe to have a stash of these cooked fish sticks ready in the freezer for reheating. They freeze beautifully and can be prepared from frozen in the oven or toaster oven at 400°F for about 18 minutes. They are a go-to quick and easy lunch in my house.

1. Preheat the oven to 450°F.
2. In a medium bowl, whisk together the eggs, mustard, and lemon juice.
3. In another bowl, whisk together the bread crumbs, thyme, dill, onion powder, and salt.
4. Dip the cod first in the egg mixture and then into the bread crumbs, coating completely and tapping off any excess.
5. Place the fish pieces on a rimmed baking sheet. Bake for 12 to 15 minutes, flipping once, until golden brown and the fish is opaque and flakes apart.
6. Meanwhile, in a small bowl, whisk together the Greek yogurt, pickle, lemon zest, and tarragon. Serve as a dipping sauce with the fish sticks.

INGREDIENT TIP: To make your own whole-grain or gluten-free bread crumbs, cut slices of bread up into cubes and allow them to sit out on the counter for a day or two. Then, pulse them in a blender or food processor and store them in a cool, dry place in a resealable bag.

Turkey and Veggie Meatballs

DF GF **NF**

SERVES 6

PREP TIME: 10 MINUTES
COOK TIME: 17 MINUTES

1 pound ground turkey

1 carrot, grated

½ onion, grated

1 medium
zucchini, grated

1 large egg, beaten

1 teaspoon
Dijon mustard

1 tablespoon
Worcestershire sauce

½ teaspoon garlic powder

1 teaspoon dried thyme

These mini veggie meatballs freeze and reheat well, so they're a great make-ahead lunch food. Serve them with steamed brown rice, toss them in vegetable broth with some chopped veggies to make a quick soup, or put them on slider buns or toasted bread rounds to make a quick sandwich.

1. Preheat the oven to 400°F.
2. In a medium bowl, combine the turkey, carrot, onion, zucchini, egg, mustard, Worcestershire sauce, garlic powder, and thyme. Mix well without overworking.
3. Using a melon baller, scoop into small meatballs and form lightly into meatballs. Place on a rimmed baking sheet.
4. Bake for about 17 minutes, until browned.

COOKING TIP: Make cleanup a snap by lining your baking sheet with foil and lightly brushing it with olive oil to prevent sticking.

Chicken Teriyaki Meatballs

DF GF **NF**

SERVES 6

PREP TIME: 10 MINUTES
COOK TIME: 17 MINUTES

1 pound ground chicken

2 scallions, both white
and green parts,
finely chopped

½ teaspoon garlic powder

1 teaspoon fresh
ginger, grated

1 large egg, beaten

1 cup coleslaw
cabbage mix or grated
green cabbage

¼ cup reduced-
sodium tamari

3 teaspoons cornstarch

2 tablespoons honey or
pure maple syrup

Try these meatballs with Cauliflower Rice (page 144) as a delicious lunch or easy family dinner. They freeze well, and since you make the sauce and meatballs separately, you can store them separately and use the teriyaki sauce as a dip or condiment instead of coating the meatballs in them.

1. Preheat the oven to 400°F.
2. In a medium bowl, combine the chicken, scallions, garlic powder, ginger, egg, and cabbage. Mix well without overworking.
3. Using a melon baller, scoop into small meatballs and form lightly into meatballs. Place on a nonstick rimmed baking sheet.
4. Bake for about 17 minutes, until browned.
5. Meanwhile, in a small saucepan, whisk together the tamari, cornstarch, honey, and ¼ cup water. Cook, stirring, on medium-high heat for about 4 minutes, until the mixture thickens. Serve the sauce either drizzled over the meatballs or on the side as a dipping sauce.

COOKING TIP: You can also make this into a slow cooker meal. Make the meatballs and arrange them in a slow cooker. Mix the sauce and, instead of cooking it on the stovetop, pour it over the meatballs in the slow cooker. Cook on low for 8 hours.

SUBSTITUTION TIP: If gluten is not an issue, you can substitute reduced-sodium soy sauce for the tamari.

Make-Ahead Ham, Egg, and Cheese Muffins

GF NF

SERVES 6

PREP TIME: 5 MINUTES
COOK TIME: 30 MINUTES

Olive oil, for greasing

6 large eggs, beaten

½ cup whole milk or non-dairy milk (see page 76)

Pinch sea salt

6 ounces ham, chopped

½ cup Cheddar cheese, grated

3 scallions, both white and green parts, finely chopped

So easy to make, easy to freeze, and easy to pack, these little muffins are perfect for little lunch boxes, a quick breakfast or dinner, or whenever you need a meal on the go. Reheat them in the microwave for a minute or so on high or serve them cold. Either way, they're tasty.

1. Preheat the oven to 350°F. Brush a 6-cup muffin tin with olive oil.
2. In a medium bowl, whisk together the eggs, milk, and salt.
3. Fold in the ham, cheese, and scallions.
4. Spoon into the prepared muffin tins and bake for about 30 minutes, until set.

COOKING TIP: Make these vegetarian by omitting the ham, or up the nutrition by grating or finely chopping veggies and sautéing them before folding them into the eggs. These are incredibly versatile.

English Muffin Pizza Bites

NF

SERVES 2

PREP TIME: 15 MINUTES
COOK TIME: 10 MINUTES

2 tablespoons
tomato paste

¼ teaspoon garlic powder

¼ teaspoon
dried oregano

1 whole-grain English
muffin, split

2 ounces mini pepperoni

¼ cup Parmesan or
mozzarella cheese, grated

These are a fun family project your toddler will love helping with. Put out dishes with toppings and allow everyone to top their own pizza. After baking, cut your toddler's pizza into small wedges for easy eating.

1. Preheat the oven to 375°F. Line a baking sheet with parchment paper.
2. In a small bowl, whisk together the tomato paste, garlic powder, oregano, and 1 teaspoon water. Spread onto the cut half of each English muffin and place the muffins on the prepared baking sheet.
3. Add the pepperoni to each muffin. Sprinkle with the cheese.
4. Bake in the preheated oven for about 10 minutes, until the cheese melts.

VARIATION TIP: Make these vegetarian by replacing the pepperoni with sautéed red peppers. Use cooked crumbled sausage, or top with crumbled bacon for variations on flavor.

Chop Salad

GF NF

SERVES 2

PREP TIME: 15 MINUTES

4 ounces boneless skinless cooked chicken, finely chopped

4 scallions, both white and green parts, finely chopped

¼ cup black olives, finely chopped

1 ounce mozzarella cheese, finely chopped

1 canned artichoke bottom, finely chopped

2 basil leaves, finely chopped

2 tablespoons apple cider vinegar

1 tablespoon freshly squeezed lemon juice

1 garlic clove, minced

1 teaspoon Dijon mustard

¼ cup extra-virgin olive oil

Pinch sea salt

The beauty of the chop salad is this: You can pretty much chop any veggies, herbs, and meats into a "salad" and top them with a quick vinaigrette or creamy dressing and you've got a quick and easily varied toddler meal. This one has Italian flavor profiles.

1. In a medium bowl, combine the chicken, scallions, olives, mozzarella, and artichokes. Mix well.
2. In a small bowl, whisk together the basil, apple cider vinegar, lemon juice, garlic, mustard, olive oil, and salt. Toss with the salad and serve.

VARIATION TIP: You can leave out the cheese and replace it with a finely chopped veggie to make this dairy-free. To make it vegetarian, replace the chicken with chopped tofu.

Corn and Baby Shrimp Salad with Dill

SERVES 2

PREP TIME: 15 MINUTES

4 ounces cooked baby shrimp, chilled

¼ cup cooked frozen corn kernels, cooled

½ red bell pepper, finely chopped

¼ avocado, chopped

3 cherry tomatoes, finely chopped

Juice of 1 lemon

Pinch sea salt

2 tablespoons extra-virgin olive oil

1 tablespoon fresh dill, chopped

This salad will keep in the fridge for up to 3 days, and you can add any soft chopped veggies you like. If you can find in-season corn on the cob, blanch the corn in boiling water for 2 minutes and then cut it from the cob with a knife. Otherwise, frozen corn is a good alternative.

1. In a medium bowl, combine the shrimp, corn, bell pepper, avocado, and cherry tomatoes.
2. In a small bowl, whisk together the lemon juice, salt, olive oil, and dill. Toss with the salad.

SUBSTITUTION TIP: If your kiddo is allergic to shellfish, which is a common allergen, you can replace the shrimp with 4 ounces of cooked, chopped chicken.

Rainbow Pepper Crustless Mini Quiches

SERVES 6

PREP TIME: 10 MINUTES
COOK TIME: 20 MINUTES

2 tablespoons extra-virgin olive oil, plus extra for greasing

½ red bell pepper, finely chopped

½ yellow bell pepper, finely chopped

½ orange bell pepper, finely chopped

1 garlic clove, minced

¼ teaspoon sea salt

6 large eggs, beaten

½ cup whole milk or non-dairy milk (see page 76)

½ cup Parmesan cheese, grated

These mini crustless quiches freeze very well, and they're delicious cold or warm so they're quite versatile. If you can't find various colors of peppers, you can always just use peppers in one color. While the result won't be as eye-catching, they'll still be delicious.

1. Preheat the oven to 350°F. Brush a 6-cup muffin tin lightly with olive oil.
2. In a large nonstick skillet, heat the olive oil on medium high until it shimmers.
3. Add the peppers, garlic, and salt, and cook, stirring occasionally, for about 4 minutes, until soft. Cool completely.
4. In large bowl, whisk together the eggs and milk. Fold in the cooled peppers and the cheese. Distribute into the prepared muffin tins.
5. Bake for 20 to 25 minutes, until they are set and the tops are lightly browned.

SUBSTITUTION TIP: If desired, you can omit the olive oil for brushing the muffin tin and use muffin tin liners instead.

Veggie Burgers with Homemade Ketchup

SERVES 4

PREP TIME: 20 MINUTES
COOK TIME: 10 MINUTES

FOR THE KETCHUP

6 ounces tomato paste

2 tablespoons apple
cider vinegar

1 teaspoon
mustard powder

½ teaspoon garlic powder

2 teaspoons
onion powder

1 tablespoon honey or
pure maple syrup

½ teaspoon sea salt

FOR THE BURGERS

1 cup cooked quinoa

½ cup cooked brown rice

¼ cup gluten-free
rolled oats

½ cup baby spinach,
finely chopped

1 carrot, peeled
and grated

1 large egg, beaten

2 tablespoons plain
Greek whole-milk yogurt

½ teaspoon sea salt

½ teaspoon
ground cumin

½ teaspoon garlic powder

½ teaspoon
onion powder

Extra-virgin olive oil,
for cooking

4 gluten-free
hamburger buns

If you're looking for an easy veggie burger, these patties will fit the bill. They freeze well (freeze them cooked and reheat them in the oven or microwave), and you can serve them alone or on slider buns for a quick burger. This is another recipe I often double or triple to build up my freezer stash. The homemade ketchup is more flavorful and lower in sugar than commercial varieties and makes about 1 cup of ketchup. You can always double or triple it, as it lasts about 4 weeks in the fridge.

TO MAKE THE KETCHUP

In a small saucepan, combine the tomato paste, vinegar, mustard powder, garlic powder, onion powder, honey, sea salt, and ¼ cup water. Simmer on medium heat, stirring, until it reaches the desired consistency. Refrigerate in an airtight container.

TO MAKE THE BURGERS

1. In a large bowl, combine the quinoa, rice, oats, spinach, and carrot.
2. In a small bowl, whisk together the egg, yogurt, salt, cumin, garlic powder, and onion powder.
3. Mix the wet ingredients with the dry. Cover and refrigerate for at least 30 minutes.
4. Form the mixture into 4 patties.
5. In a large, nonstick skillet, heat the olive oil on medium high until it shimmers.
6. Cook the patties about 4 minutes per side, flipping once, until browned. Serve on the hamburger buns, topped with ketchup.

SUBSTITUTION TIP: For a spicier ketchup, add a pinch cayenne or ½ teaspoon of chili powder. To make this vegan and dairy-free, replace the Greek yogurt with vegan mayonnaise.

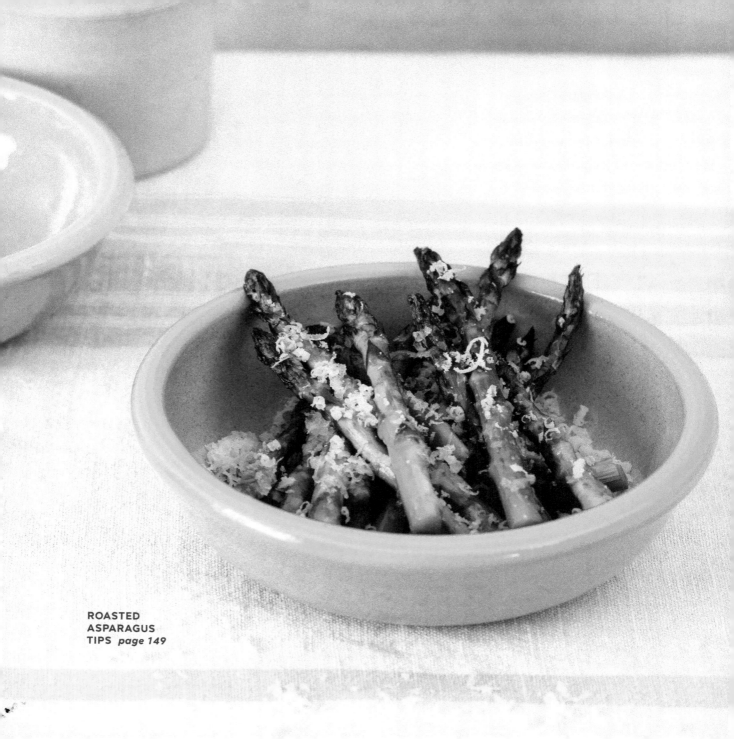

ROASTED
ASPARAGUS
TIPS *page 149*

8

SIDES

The best sides for your little ones are packed with nutritious veggies to add valuable vitamins and minerals to your child's diet. Many people rely strongly on grain-based side dishes to fill out a plate, and while a small serving of grains is fine, the most nutritious meals have a healthy helping of colorful vegetables as a side dish. Choose veggies across the spectrum of colors to ensure your toddler is getting all of the nutrients she needs.

Cauliflower Rice

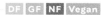

SERVES 6

PREP TIME: 10 MINUTES
COOK TIME: 5 MINUTES

1 cauliflower head, cut from fibrous stems and separated into florets

2 tablespoons extra-virgin olive oil

Pinch kosher salt

I love cauliflower rice. It's a great way to add extra veggies to your toddler's diet, and it's really versatile. Plus, it's super easy to make a batch and it cooks more quickly than regular rice. You can substitute cauliflower rice in any of the recipes in this book that call for rice.

1. In a food processor, pulse the florets of cauliflower for 15 to 25 (1-second) pulses until the cauliflower resembles rice.
2. In a large, nonstick skillet, heat the olive oil on medium high until it shimmers.
3. Add the cauliflower and cook for about 5 minutes, until tender. Season with the salt.

INGREDIENT TIP: You can also grate the cauliflower on a box grater or by using the grater attachment of your food processor.

Veggie Noodles (Zoodles)

SERVES 2

PREP TIME: 10 MINUTES
COOK TIME: 5 MINUTES

1 medium zucchini

2 tablespoons extra-virgin olive oil

Pinch kosher salt

Veggie noodles are another great way to add more vegetables to your toddler's diet. While the easiest way to make the noodles is to use a spiralizer, you can also create them by using a vegetable peeler to cut them into long strips, and then use a sharp knife to cut the strips lengthwise to the desired width. A julienne peeler is another easy way to make noodles if you don't have a spiralizer.

1. Using a spiralizer or vegetable peeler and knife, prep the zucchini into spaghetti-shaped strips.
2. In a large, nonstick skillet, heat the olive oil on medium high until it shimmers.
3. Add the zucchini and cook for about 5 minutes, until tender. Season with salt.

SUBSTITUTION TIP: Some veggies are more suited to making into noodles than others. Other good choices are carrots, sweet potato, yellow squash, and acorn or butternut squash.

Sautéed Citrus Spinach

SERVES 4

PREP TIME: 10 MINUTES
COOK TIME: 9 MINUTES

2 tablespoons extra-virgin olive oil

2 cups baby spinach, finely chopped

1 garlic clove, minced

Juice of ½ orange

Pinch kosher salt

For toddlers, it's important you cut greens up into very small pieces so they are easy to eat. For tougher greens like kale and Swiss chard, cut out the tough, fibrous stems and then use a sharp knife to cut the greens up into very small pieces that your toddler can easily chew and swallow.

1. In a large, nonstick skillet, heat the olive oil on medium high until it shimmers.
2. Add the spinach and cook, stirring occasionally, for about 5 minutes, until soft.
3. Add the garlic and cook, stirring constantly, for 30 seconds.
4. Add the orange juice. Cook for about 3 minutes more, stirring, until the liquid reduces by half. Season with salt.

SUBSTITUTION TIP: Other greens will work well here, too, including spinach, collard greens, mustard greens, or beet greens.

Zucchini Cakes

SERVES 4

PREP TIME: 10 MINUTES
COOK TIME: 20 MINUTES

1 medium
zucchini, grated

1 teaspoon kosher salt

1 scallion, both white
and green parts,
finely chopped

½ teaspoon garlic powder

1 large egg, beaten

1 tablespoon nondairy
milk (see page 76)

½ teaspoon
Dijon mustard

½ cup whole-wheat flour

These zucchini cakes are quick and easy, and they make a tasty side. Serve them with a dollop of plain Greek yogurt and some chopped chives. Salting the zucchini ahead of time helps remove some of the bitter juices it contains and gives it a drier texture that allows it to bake better.

1. Preheat the oven to 400°F.
2. Place a colander in the sink and add the zucchini. Sprinkle the salt evenly over the top. Allow to drain for 10 minutes. Rinse and pat dry with paper towels, pressing out any excess liquid as you do.
3. In a large bowl, add the zucchini and the scallion.
4. In a small bowl, whisk together the garlic powder, egg, milk, mustard, and flour.
5. Toss with the zucchini. Form the mixture into 4 cakes and place on a nonstick rimmed baking sheet.
6. Bake for about 20 minutes, flipping once, until golden.

SUBSTITUTION TIP: You can also use sweet potatoes or any type of grated winter squash in these cakes. To make them gluten-free, use a gluten-free all-purpose flour in place of the whole-wheat flour.

Smashed Cauliflower

SERVES 4 TO 6

PREP TIME: 10 MINUTES
COOK TIME: 10 MINUTES

1 cauliflower head, cut
from fibrous stems and
broken into florets

½ teaspoon sea salt

2 tablespoons unsalted
butter, melted

¼ cup whole milk or non-
dairy milk (see page 76)

2 tablespoons fresh
chives, chopped

¼ teaspoon freshly
ground black pepper

This is a slightly less starchy, slightly more nutritious version of smashed potatoes. Cauliflower is an excellent source of vitamin C and fiber. The cauliflower yields a similar texture but has fewer natural sugars than potatoes do. It makes a great side, and it also freezes well.

1. In a large pot, cover the cauliflower florets with water. Add the salt. Cover and bring to a simmer on medium-high heat for about 10 minutes, until the cauliflower is tender.
2. Drain the cauliflower and return it to the dry pot.
3. Add the butter, milk, chives, and pepper. Using a potato masher, mash the cauliflower until it is mostly smooth and blended.

SUBSTITUTION TIP: For nondairy and vegan, you can replace the butter with either vegan butter or olive oil and replace the milk with a nondairy milk of your choice.

Roasted Asparagus Tips

SERVES 4

PREP TIME: 10 MINUTES
COOK TIME: 15 MINUTES

1 asparagus bunch,
tips trimmed and stalks
reserved for another use

2 tablespoons extra-
virgin olive oil

¼ teaspoon kosher salt

Pinch freshly ground
black pepper

¼ cup Parmesan cheese,
grated (optional)

The tips of asparagus are tender and easy for toddlers to eat. Save the stalks and use them in another recipe, such as in asparagus soup or in a stir-fry, or serve them to the adults as a dinner side. This is best with the thin asparagus that are available early in the season.

1. Preheat the oven to 425°F.
2. In a small bowl, toss the asparagus tips with the olive oil, salt, and pepper. Spread in a single layer on a rimmed baking sheet.
3. Bake for 12 to 15 minutes, stirring once or twice, until the asparagus tips are browned and tender.
4. Sprinkle with the cheese (if using).

SUBSTITUTION TIP: Cheese is optional here so you can easily make these asparagus tips vegan and dairy-free.

Roasted Spiced Acorn Squash

SERVES 4

PREP TIME: 10 MINUTES
COOK TIME: 20 MINUTES

1 cup acorn
squash, cubed

1 tablespoon extra-virgin
olive oil

¼ teaspoon ground
cinnamon

⅛ teaspoon
ground nutmeg

¼ teaspoon
ground ginger

¼ teaspoon kosher salt

Many grocery stores now offer uncooked acorn or butternut squash already cut into cubes. If you can find them, your prep time will be even quicker. The warm spices complement the slightly sweet, earthy flavor of the squash.

1. Preheat the oven to 400°F.
2. In a small bowl, toss the squash with the olive oil, cinnamon, nutmeg, and ginger. Spread in a single layer on a rimmed baking sheet.
3. Bake for about 20 minutes, stirring once or twice, until the squash is browned and tender. Season with the salt.

SUBSTITUTION TIP: This is also a great way to prepare cubed sweet potatoes or carrots. The spice blend can remain the same, or you can use more savory spices, such as ¼ teaspoon each of ground coriander and ground cumin.

Orange-Maple Roasted Carrots

SERVES 4

PREP TIME: 10 MINUTES
COOK TIME: 20 MINUTES

1 tablespoon coconut
oil, melted

1 tablespoon pure
maple syrup

½ teaspoon fresh
ginger, grated

Zest of ½ orange

3 carrots, peeled and cut
into cubes

¼ teaspoon kosher salt

This simple roasted carrot dish is warm and satisfying with hints of maple and ginger. It makes an excellent side dish or snack, and if you double or triple the recipe you can use it to feed a crowd.

1. Preheat the oven to 400°F. Line a rimmed baking sheet with parchment paper.
2. In a small bowl, whisk together the coconut oil, maple syrup, ginger, and orange zest.
3. Toss with the carrots and spread in a single layer on the prepared baking sheet.
4. Bake for 15 to 20 minutes, until the carrots are tender.
5. Season with salt.

SUBSTITUTION TIP: If you're not worried about this being vegan or dairy-free, you can replace the maple syrup with honey and the coconut oil with unsalted butter.

Brown Rice with Bell Peppers

SERVES 4

PREP TIME: 10 MINUTES
COOK TIME: 10 MINUTES

2 tablespoons extra-virgin olive oil

¼ onion, finely chopped

½ yellow bell pepper, finely chopped

½ red bell pepper, finely chopped

1 garlic clove, minced

1 cup cooked brown rice

¼ cup unsalted vegetable broth

½ teaspoon dried thyme

Salt

Freshly ground black pepper

For this recipe, you can use any cooked whole grain, such as farro or quinoa. I recommend brown rice because it's easy to find precooked at the grocery store. If you choose to precook the whole grains yourself, do so according to the package instructions and store it in the freezer in ½-cup servings so you have it readily available for quick recipes throughout the week.

1. In a large, nonstick skillet, heat the olive oil on medium high until it shimmers.
2. Add the onion and bell peppers and cook for about 5 minutes, stirring occasionally, until soft.
3. Add the garlic and cook, stirring constantly, for 30 seconds.
4. Add the rice, vegetable broth, and thyme. Bring to a simmer and cook, stirring, for 3 minutes. Season with salt and pepper.

SUBSTITUTION TIP: This is a versatile dish; you can switch the grain, vegetables, or spices to your own desires. You can also add ¼ cup of peas when you add the vegetable broth for a nice bit of vegetable protein and color.

Roasted Beets with Tarragon

SERVES 4

PREP TIME: 10 MINUTES
COOK TIME: 40 MINUTES

**2 golden beets, peeled
and cut into ½-inch cubes**

**1 tablespoon extra-virgin
olive oil**

**1 teaspoon dried
tarragon**

Zest of ½ orange

Salt

**Freshly ground
black pepper**

Beets take a bit longer to roast than other vegetables, but the result is worth it. The end product is tender, earthy, slightly sweet, and delicious. Fortunately, most of the time is passive—you can put the beets in the oven and do something else while they roast. I use golden beets because they don't stain like red beets do. These will keep in the freezer for up to 6 months or in the fridge for up to 5 days.

1. Preheat the oven to 400°F. Line a rimmed baking sheet with parchment paper.
2. In a medium bowl, toss the beets with the olive oil, tarragon, and orange zest. Spread in a single layer on the prepared baking sheet.
3. Bake for 30 to 40 minutes, stirring once or twice, until the beets are tender. Season with salt and pepper.

SUBSTITUTION TIP: This recipe is a great go-to for any dense root vegetable, such as turnips, sweet potatoes, or celeriac.

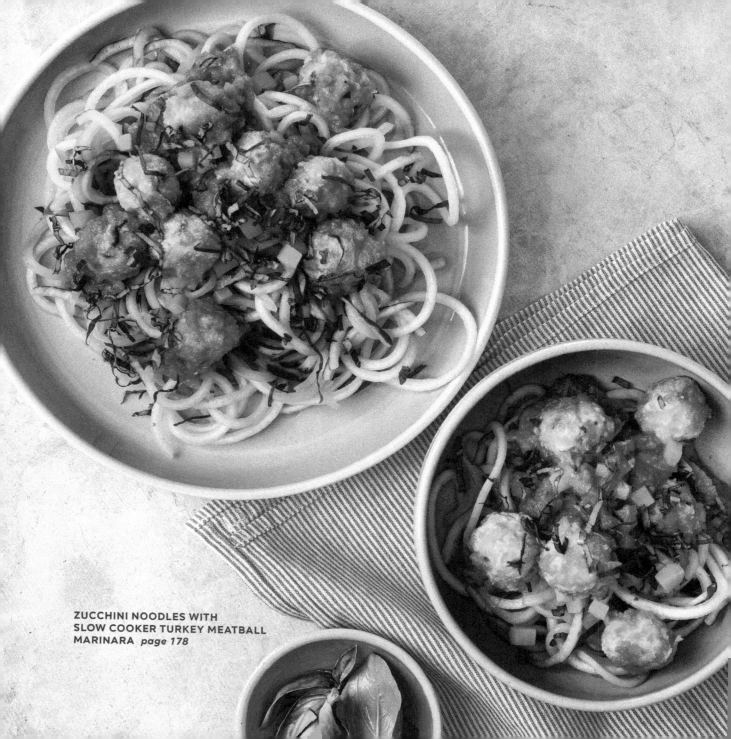

ZUCCHINI NOODLES WITH
SLOW COOKER TURKEY MEATBALL
MARINARA *page 178*

9

FAMILY DINNERS

I understand that parents are busy, and making one meal for the family and another for your toddler creates an excessive workload. Plus, introducing your toddler to the foods your family eats as soon as possible not only lightens your load, it also ensures your toddler is exposed to a wide array of foods. These dinners are great for the entire family. Where you may need to make adaptations for your toddler, it's called out in the recipe. For example, sometimes you'll want to separate your toddler's portion before you add spicier ingredients.

Pumpkin Soup

SERVES 4 TO 6

PREP TIME: 10 MINUTES
COOK TIME: 15 MINUTES

2 tablespoons extra-virgin olive oil

1 onion, finely chopped

3 garlic cloves, minced

2 (14-ounce) cans pumpkin purée

6 cups unsalted vegetable broth

1 teaspoon dried sage

1 (14-ounce) can coconut milk

1 teaspoon sea salt

Freshly ground black pepper

½ cup pepitas (optional)

This simple vegetarian soup is warming and delicious, and it can feed the whole family without any modifications for your toddler because, while it has a lovely herb and spice profile, it isn't particularly spicy. It also freezes well, which means it's great in big batches. If you double your recipe, you can cook once and eat at least twice, which is a huge time-saver.

1. In a large pot, heat the olive oil on medium high until it shimmers. Add the onion and cook, stirring occasionally, for about 5 minutes, until softened.
2. Add the garlic and cook, stirring constantly, for 30 seconds.
3. Add the pumpkin purée, vegetable broth, and sage. Bring to a boil, stirring occasionally, until it simmers. Reduce the heat to medium low and simmer for 5 minutes, stirring occasionally.
4. Add the coconut milk and stir until it is blended.
5. Using an immersion blender, blender, or food processor, purée the soup.
6. Taste and season with salt and pepper. Serve with the pepitas as garnish (if using).

SUBSTITUTION TIP: For very young toddlers, leave off the pepitas and serve the soup plain, or offer with crumbled crackers as garnish. You can also substitute steamed sweet potato or squash for the pumpkin. To do this, simmer two peeled and chopped sweet potatoes or squash in the vegetable broth in step 3 and increase simmering time for about 10 minutes, or until the vegetables are soft.

Weeknight Chicken Soup

DF GF NF

SERVES 4 TO 6

PREP TIME: 10 MINUTES
COOK TIME: 20 MINUTES

2 tablespoons extra-
virgin olive oil

1 onion, finely chopped

1 celery stalk,
finely chopped

2 carrots, peeled
and chopped

1 pound boneless,
skinless chicken breasts
or thighs, cut into
½-inch pieces

6 cups unsalted
vegetable or
chicken broth

1 zucchini, finely chopped

1 red bell pepper,
finely chopped

1 teaspoon garlic powder

1 teaspoon dried
rosemary

2 cups fresh or
frozen peas

1 teaspoon sea salt

Freshly ground
black pepper

This is a versatile soup you can make in big batches. Once you've made the soup, you can add a starch, such as cooked brown rice, cooked quinoa, or cooked noodles to the soup if desired, or eat it as is—a delicious chicken and vegetable soup.

1. In a large pot, heat the olive oil on medium high until it shimmers. Add the onion, celery, and carrots and cook, stirring occasionally, for about 5 minutes, until the veggies are soft.

2. Add the chicken and cook, stirring occasionally, about 5 minutes more, until cooked through.

3. Add the vegetable broth, zucchini, bell pepper, garlic powder, and rosemary. Bring to a simmer, stirring occasionally. Reduce the heat to medium low and simmer, stirring occasionally, for about 10 minutes more, until the vegetables are tender.

4. Stir in the peas and cook until heated through, 3 to 4 minutes more.

5. Taste and season with the salt and pepper.

COOKING TIP: Making your own broth is easy, especially in the slow cooker. I like to save trimmings (including peels) from carrots, celery, mushrooms, onions, garlic, and fresh herbs in a resealable bag in my freezer. When I have a full 2-gallon ziptop bag, I dump the vegetables into the slow cooker, add a few peppercorns, and cover the trimmings with water. Cover the slow cooker and cook on low for 8 hours. Strain and freeze in 1-cup servings in the freezer. For poultry broth, I add about a pound of meaty chicken bones, such as wings, necks, or backs to the frozen veggies and simmer the stock for 12 to 24 hours.

Chicken Tortilla Soup

SERVES 4 TO 6

PREP TIME: 10 MINUTES
COOK TIME: 20 MINUTES

This soup can be a bit spicy, so I recommend scooping out your toddler portions before adding the canned chopped chile peppers and chili powder at the end. Depending on food allergies, you can also choose to leave off any of the garnishes or add your own.

2 tablespoons extra-virgin olive oil

1 onion, finely chopped

1 pound boneless, skinless chicken breasts or thighs, cut into ½-inch pieces

4 garlic cloves, minced

5 cups unsalted chicken broth

1 (14-ounce) can crushed tomatoes

1 (14-ounce) can black beans, drained

1 teaspoon dried oregano

1 teaspoon ground cumin

1 teaspoon sea salt

Freshly ground black pepper

1 (4.5-ounce) can chopped green chiles, drained

1 teaspoon chili powder

2 whole-wheat or corn tortillas, toasted and chopped into small pieces

Lime wedges, for garnish (optional)

Grated Monterey Jack cheese, for garnish (optional)

Fresh cilantro, chopped, for garnish (optional)

Scallions, both white and green parts, thinly sliced, for garnish (optional)

Avocado, diced, for garnish (optional)

1. In a large pot, heat the olive oil on medium high until it shimmers. Add the onion and cook, stirring occasionally, for about 5 minutes, until softened.

2. Add the chicken and cook, stirring occasionally, about 5 minutes more, until the chicken is cooked through.

3. Add the garlic and cook, stirring constantly, for 30 seconds.

4. Add the chicken broth, tomatoes with their juices, black beans, oregano, and cumin. Bring to a simmer. Reduce the heat to medium and cook, stirring occasionally, for 8 minutes.

5. Taste and season with the salt and pepper.

6. Separate a toddler portion and set aside.

7. To the remaining soup, add the chopped green chiles and chili powder. Cook until the chiles are warmed through, 1 or 2 minutes more.

8. Serve topped with the toasted tortilla strips and any other garnishes you choose.

COOKING TIP: To toast the tortillas, heat them in a single layer in a 350°F oven until crisp, about 7 minutes. For toddlers, make sure the strips are crumbled or cut very small.

Slow Cooker Bone Broth

`DF` `GF` `NF`

MAKES 8 TO 10 CUPS

PREP TIME: 10 MINUTES
COOK TIME: 12 TO 48 HOURS

2 pounds organic beef
or poultry bones

1 onion, quartered

3 garlic cloves

1 carrot, roughly chopped

1 celery stalk

1 thyme or rosemary sprig

6 peppercorns

1 tablespoon
apple cider vinegar

Water to fill a 4- to 6-quart
slow cooker

This nutrient-rich stock is made so simple in the slow cooker there's no excuse not to make it. It boosts the immune system, improves digestion, and builds strong bones, hair, and nails. Grass-fed, organic animal bones are the way to go for this recipe—you can store bones in a resealable plastic bag in the freezer until you have enough for this recipe.

1. Combine all the ingredients in the slow cooker. Cover and set on low.
2. Cook for a minimum of 12 hours and up to 48 hours for beef bones or up to 24 hours for poultry bones.
3. Strain out the solids and discard. Refrigerate overnight and skim off the fat.
4. Keep in 1-cup servings in the freezer for up to 6 months.

COOKING TIP: Bone broth is the perfect base for any soup. Add in quinoa and shredded chicken or blended vegetables for an easy weeknight meal.

New England Clam Chowder

SERVES 4 TO 6

PREP TIME: 10 MINUTES
COOK TIME: 20 MINUTES

4 pepper bacon
slices, chopped

1 onion, finely chopped

1 fennel bulb,
finely chopped

1 carrot, peeled
and chopped

1 red bell pepper,
finely chopped

2 garlic cloves, minced

3 tablespoons all-
purpose flour

6 cups vegetable or
chicken broth

2 (6.5-ounce) cans baby
clams, undrained

1 pound baby red
potatoes, quartered

1 teaspoon dried
tarragon

¼ cup whole milk or non-
dairy milk (see page 76)

1 teaspoon sea salt

2 tablespoons fresh
fennel fronds, chopped

This is a delicious warming soup your whole family will love. Fennel adds a subtle anise flavor that perfectly complements the clams, and the soup is hearty enough that it's a meal by itself. You can also substitute other fish for the clams, such as halibut or cod, for a fish chowder.

1. In a large pot, cook the pepper bacon for about 5 minutes on medium high, stirring occasionally, until browned. Using a slotted spoon, remove the bacon from the fat and set aside.
2. In the bacon fat, cook the onion, fennel, carrot, and bell pepper for about 5 minutes, stirring occasionally, until the vegetables begin to soften.
3. Add the garlic, and cook for 30 seconds, stirring constantly.
4. Add the flour and cook, stirring constantly, for 2 minutes.
5. Add the vegetable broth, scraping any browned bits from the bottom of the pot with the side of a spoon. Add the clams, potatoes, and tarragon. Bring to a boil and reduce to a simmer. Cook, stirring occasionally, for about 10 minutes, until the potatoes are softened.
6. Stir in the milk. Taste and season as needed with the salt. Stir in the fennel fronds and the reserved bacon. Serve immediately.

SUBSTITUTION TIP: It's easy to make this soup vegetarian; substitute 2 (14-ounce) cans of drained corn for the clams to make a tasty corn chowder and omit the bacon. You can also make the soup dairy-free by using a nondairy milk.

Pasta e Fagioli Soup

SERVES 4 TO 6

PREP TIME: 10 MINUTES
COOK TIME: 20 MINUTES

2 tablespoons extra-virgin olive oil

1 onion, finely chopped

1 red bell pepper, finely chopped

1 pound bulk sweet Italian sausage

3 garlic cloves, minced

6 cups unsalted chicken broth

1 (14-ounce) can pinto beans, drained

1 (14-ounce) can chopped tomatoes

1 teaspoon dried Italian herbs

1½ cups dried elbow macaroni

1 teaspoon sea salt

Freshly ground black pepper

Pasta e Fagioli is a hearty, thick pasta and bean soup. This version also features tasty sweet Italian sausage, which pumps up the flavor without adding heat. If you prefer a spicier soup, you can remove your toddler portion and then add a pinch of red pepper flakes. Simmer the soup with the red pepper flakes for about 5 minutes before serving to infuse the flavor.

1. In a large pot, heat the olive oil on medium high until it shimmers. Add the onion and bell pepper and cook, stirring occasionally, for about 5 minutes, until the vegetables soften.
2. Add the sausage and cook, crumbling with a spoon, until it is browned.
3. Add the garlic and cook, stirring constantly, for 30 seconds.
4. Add the chicken broth, pinto beans, tomatoes with their juices, and Italian herbs. Bring to a boil, stirring occasionally.
5. Add the elbow macaroni. Cook, stirring occasionally, for about 8 minutes more, until the pasta is al dente.
6. Season with the salt and pepper. Serve.

COOKING TIP: If desired, garnish each bowl of soup with 2 tablespoons of grated Parmesan cheese.

Spaghetti Squash Primavera

SERVES 4 TO 6

PREP TIME: 10 MINUTES
COOK TIME: 40 MINUTES

2 whole spaghetti squash, halved lengthwise and seeded

6 tablespoons extra-virgin olive oil, divided

2 carrots, peeled and chopped

1 onion, chopped

1 red bell pepper, chopped

2 zucchini, peeled and chopped

3 garlic cloves, minced

Juice of 1 lemon

¼ cup chicken broth

¼ cup heavy cream

1 pint cherry tomatoes, quartered

½ cup Parmesan cheese, grated

½ teaspoon sea salt

Freshly ground black pepper

¼ cup fresh basil, chopped

Primavera is a sauce made from seasonal vegetables. Traditionally served with pasta, this version uses spaghetti squash. The spaghetti squash takes a bit to cook, but you can make it ahead and store it in the fridge for up to 5 days, so it's great to roast on the weekend and pull out for a busy weeknight meal.

1. Preheat the oven to 450°F.
2. Brush the cut sides of the spaghetti squash with 4 tablespoons of the olive oil and place them cut-side down on a rimmed baking sheet. Bake until soft, about 30 to 40 minutes. Cool slightly and then use the tines of a fork to scrape the flesh from the rind into spaghetti-like strands.
3. In a large pot, heat the remaining 2 tablespoons of olive oil on medium high until it shimmers.
4. Add the carrots, onion, bell pepper, and zucchini and cook for 5 to 7 minutes, stirring occasionally, until the vegetables soften.
5. Add the garlic and cook, stirring constantly, for 30 seconds.
6. Add the lemon juice and chicken broth, using the side of a spoon to scrape any browned bits from the bottom of the pan. Bring to a simmer. Reduce the heat to medium low and simmer until the liquid reduces by half, about 3 to 4 minutes.
7. Stir in the heavy cream. Bring to a simmer.
8. Stir in the cherry tomatoes and spaghetti squash. Cook until the tomatoes and squash are warmed, 2 to 3 minutes more. Sprinkle with the Parmesan cheese, taste, and season with the salt and pepper.
9. Serve garnished with the chopped basil.

SUBSTITUTION TIP: To make this vegan and dairy-free, replace the heavy cream with any nondairy milk and omit the Parmesan cheese.

Zucchini Lasagna Muffins

 GF NF V

SERVES 6 TO 8

PREP TIME: 10 MINUTES
COOK TIME: 20 MINUTES

2 tablespoons extra-virgin olive oil, plus extra for greasing

1 onion, finely chopped

3 garlic cloves, minced

1 (14-ounce) can crushed tomatoes, drained

1 (14-ounce) can tomato sauce

2 teaspoons dried Italian seasoning

½ teaspoon sea salt

1 medium zucchini, cut into ¼-inch slices

2 cups cottage cheese

6 ounces Swiss cheese, grated

These little lasagnas freeze well, so you can make a double batch and have a second meal later in the week (or another week). You'll want to grease your muffin tins well to prevent sticking, and be sure you thinly and evenly slice the zucchini. If you have a mandoline, slicing to ¼-inch thickness is fast and easy.

1. Preheat the oven to 450°F. Grease a 12-cup muffin tin with olive oil.
2. In a large saucepan, heat the olive oil until it shimmers. Add the onions and cook, stirring occasionally, for about 5 minutes, until soft.
3. Add the garlic and cook, stirring constantly, for 30 seconds.
4. Add the tomatoes, tomato sauce, and Italian seasoning. Bring to a simmer and reduce the heat. Simmer for 5 minutes. Taste and season with the salt.
5. In the muffin cups, spread a layer of the sauce on the bottom. Top with zucchini slices to fully cover the sauce. Add a tablespoon of cottage cheese and a tablespoon of the Swiss cheese to each cup. Add another layer of sauce, zucchini, cottage cheese, and Swiss cheese. Top with slices of zucchini, more sauce, and top with shredded cheese.
6. Bake for 20 to 30 minutes, until brown and bubbly.

SUBSTITUTION TIP: You can make this vegan and dairy-free by substituting a tofu-based soft cheese for the cottage cheese and a grated vegan cheese for the Swiss cheese.

Mac 'n' Cheese 'n' Peas

NF V

SERVES 4 TO 6

PREP TIME: 10 MINUTES
COOK TIME: 20 MINUTES

2 tablespoons extra-virgin olive oil

1 onion, finely chopped

1 butternut squash, peeled, seeded, and cut into ½-inch cubes

1 cup vegetable broth

1 cup whole milk

2 tablespoons unsalted butter

2 tablespoons cream cheese, cut into pieces

1 cup grated cheese (I like a combination that includes ¼ cup sharp Cheddar, ½ cup medium Cheddar, and ¼ cup Swiss cheese)

2 cups fresh or frozen peas, warmed on the stove top or in the microwave and drained

2 cups whole-wheat or gluten-free elbow macaroni, cooked according to package directions and drained

½ teaspoon sea salt

1 tablespoon unsalted butter

1 cup whole-grain or gluten-free bread crumbs

Mac 'n' cheese is a traditional comfort food that kids love. It's something moms have been feeding to their children for decades, and Julian for one is a big fan. This version gets a healthy makeover with either whole-grain or gluten-free macaroni and a butternut-squash-based sauce instead of a roux-based (flour and fat) sauce. It's still cheesy and delicious, but so much more nutritious than the traditional version.

1. In a large pot, heat the olive oil on medium high until it shimmers. Reduce the heat to medium low, add the onions and cook for about 10 minutes, stirring occasionally, until browned. Remove the onions from the pot and set aside.

2. In the same pot, add the squash and vegetable broth, scraping any of the browned bits of onion from the bottom of the pan with the side of a spoon. Bring to a boil on medium high. Cover and simmer until the squash is soft, about 7 minutes.

3. While the squash simmers, in a small saucepan combine the milk, butter, and cream cheese. Cook, whisking, until the butter and cream cheese have melted and the mixture is smooth.

4. Drain the squash and transfer to a blender or food processor along with the onions and milk mixture. Blend until smooth. Return to the pot and stir in the cheese until it is melted and smooth. Add the peas and pasta. Stir to blend. Season with the salt.

5. In a medium nonstick sauté pan, heat the butter on medium high until it bubbles. Add the bread crumbs. Cook, stirring constantly for 2 to 3 minutes, until they are toasted.

6. Serve the macaroni garnished with the toasted bread crumbs.

SUBSTITUTION TIP: When you add the peas, you can stir in any other heated vegetables, such as steamed broccoli.

Cod and Zucchini Cakes with Lemon-Yogurt Dipping Sauce

GF NF

SERVES 4 TO 6

PREP TIME: 10 MINUTES
COOK TIME: 30 MINUTES

FOR THE COD CAKES

1½ pounds cod, cut into ½-inch cubes

2 small zucchini, grated

2 teaspoons fresh dill, chopped

1 teaspoon lemon zest

1 teaspoon garlic powder

½ cup almond flour

1 tablespoon coconut flour

3 large eggs, beaten

½ onion, grated

FOR THE SAUCE

½ cup plain whole-milk yogurt

Juice of 1 lemon

1 teaspoon fresh dill, chopped

These are great for meals, or you can make a bigger batch and feed the whole family. Steaming the cod ahead of time makes it soft enough and allows these fish cakes to cook quickly. Almond flour replaces wheat here, so the recipe is gluten-free.

TO MAKE THE COD CAKES

1. Preheat the oven to 350°F. Line a baking sheet with parchment paper.
2. In a small saucepan fitted with a steamer insert, bring 1 inch of water to a boil.
3. Add the cod to the steamer basket. Cover and simmer until the cod is opaque, about 5 to 10 minutes.
4. Chop the cod into small pieces (or flake it with a fork) and transfer it to a small bowl.
5. Add the zucchini, dill, lemon zest, garlic powder, almond flour, coconut flour, eggs, and onion to the bowl. Gently fold to combine.
6. Form into ½-inch balls and place on the prepared baking sheet. Gently flatten.
7. Bake for about 20 minutes, until the cakes are golden brown.

TO MAKE THE SAUCE

In a small bowl, whisk together the yogurt, lemon juice, and dill. Serve with the cod cakes.

SUBSTITUTION TIP: You can use any white fish as a substitute here. You can also use salmon, although you'll want to change the flavor profile a bit. For the salmon, replace the dill in both the cakes and the sauce with an equal amount of chopped fresh tarragon, and change the lemon juice in the sauce to fresh-squeezed orange juice.

Parchment Cod with Veggies

`GF` `NF`

SERVES 4

PREP TIME: 10 MINUTES
COOK TIME: 20 MINUTES

4 (4-ounce) cod fillets, bones removed

2 cups fresh or frozen peas or frozen peas and carrots

4 large fresh thyme sprigs

4 tablespoons unsalted butter

½ cup unsalted vegetable or chicken broth

Sea salt

Freshly ground black pepper

Cooking fish in parchment (or foil) packets keeps it nice and moist as it cooks, while gently steaming the vegetables. You can use the oven, or in the summer, cook them on indirect heat on your gas or charcoal grill. Parchment paper works in temperatures up to about 400°F.

1. Preheat the oven to 400°F.
2. Lay each piece of parchment paper on a rimmed baking sheet.
3. In the center of each piece, place the cod, skin-side up.
4. Spread ½ cup of peas on the top of each piece of cod.
5. Top each with a sprig of thyme, and place dots of butter (1 tablespoon for each packet) evenly over the top of the cod and veggies.
6. Fold the parchment into packets, but don't seal the top. Carefully pour the vegetable broth into the packets. Fold at the top to seal.
7. Bake until the fish is flaky and tender, about 18 to 20 minutes. Season with salt and pepper.

SUBSTITUTION TIP: This is also a great preparation for halibut, salmon, or trout.

Maple and Soy Salmon

DF GF **NF**

SERVES 4

PREP TIME: 5 MINUTES
COOK TIME: 7 MINUTES

1 cup pure maple syrup

¼ cup tamari

Juice of 1 orange

4 (4- to 6-ounce) salmon fillets, bones removed

Tamari is a gluten-free soy sauce substitute that tastes just like soy sauce. You can find it in the Asian foods section at the grocery store. If gluten isn't an issue, you can replace it with regular soy sauce or reduced-sodium soy sauce. Serve this with the Sautéed Citrus Spinach (page 146), Roasted Asparagus Tips (page 149), or Roasted Spiced Acorn Squash (page 150) for a tasty family meal.

1. Preheat the broiler on high.
2. On a rimmed baking pan, whisk together the maple syrup, tamari, and orange juice.
3. Place the salmon in the marinade, flesh-side down for 5 minutes.
4. Remove the salmon from the marinade and transfer it, flesh-side up, to a broiling pan.
5. Broil the salmon for about 7 minutes, until it is opaque and flakes with a fork.

COOKING TIP: You can easily remove pin bones with tweezers. Place the salmon under a bright light source to find the pin bones. You can also use a magnifying glass if you are concerned you have missed some.

Salmon Burgers with Citrus Dill Aioli

DF NF

SERVES 4

PREP TIME: 5 MINUTES
COOK TIME: 7 MINUTES

1 pound cooked skinless, boneless salmon, flaked or finely chopped

1 large egg, beaten

½ cup almond flour

4 scallions, both white and green parts, finely chopped

1 teaspoon orange zest

2 tablespoons fresh dill, chopped and divided

½ teaspoon sea salt

¼ teaspoon freshly ground black pepper

2 tablespoons extra-virgin olive oil

¼ cup mayonnaise

Juice of 1 lime

Juice of ½ lemon

4 whole-grain or gluten-free hamburger buns, toasted

If you like a good burger, then you'll enjoy these tasty salmon patties. You can serve them on gluten-free or whole-grain hamburger buns, make them half the size and serve them in a lettuce wrap, or just serve them as a main dish with the aioli for dipping. Use leftover cooked salmon or canned. If using canned, be sure to drain the salmon really well before using to prevent excessive moisture in the burgers.

1. In a small bowl, combine the salmon, egg, almond flour, scallions, orange zest, 1 tablespoon of dill, salt, and pepper. Mix well and form into 4 patties.
2. In a large, nonstick skillet, heat the olive oil on medium high until it shimmers.
3. Add the patties and cook for about 4 minutes per side, flipping once, until cooked through and browned.
4. In a small bowl, whisk together the mayonnaise, lime juice, lemon juice, and the remaining 1 tablespoon of dill.
5. Spread on the toasted buns and top with the salmon.

SUBSTITUTION TIP: You can also make a shrimp patty burger for fish allergies. Substitute 1 pound of finely chopped baby shrimp for the salmon.

Tuna Melts

NF

PREP TIME: 5 MINUTES
COOK TIME: 5 MINUTES

¼ cup mayonnaise

2 tablespoons freshly squeezed orange juice

Zest of ½ orange

1 teaspoon Dijon mustard

1 tablespoon fresh tarragon, chopped

Pinch sea salt

1 cup fresh peas

3 scallions, both white and green parts, finely chopped

1 carrot, peeled and grated

2 (5-ounce) cans water-packed tuna, drained

4 whole-grain or gluten-free bread slices, toasted

1 cup Cheddar cheese, grated

You may have heard that fish and cheese never go together, but the tuna melt proves that all rules are made to be broken. This is a fast classic that is so delicious and easy. Serve it with soup (the Pumpkin Soup (page 156) is an especially good choice) or have it as a quick dinner with a side of steamed veggies.

1. Preheat the broiler on high and place the rack 6 to 8 inches from the broiler.
2. In a small bowl, whisk together the mayonnaise, orange juice, orange zest, mustard, tarragon, and salt.
3. Fold in the peas, scallions, carrot, and tuna.
4. Place the toasted bread on a rimmed baking sheet. Top with the tuna salad mixture and sprinkle the cheese over the top.
5. Broil for about 4 minutes, until the cheese is bubbly and starts to brown.

SUBSTITUTION TIP: For people with fish allergies, substitute flaked canned crab meat (drained) for the tuna.

Chicken Quesadillas with Corn and Bell Pepper Salsa

NF

SERVES 4

PREP TIME: 10 MINUTES
COOK TIME: 10 MINUTES

4 tablespoons extra-virgin olive oil, divided

8 whole-wheat or corn tortillas

1 cup Monterey Jack cheese or Mexican cheese blend, grated

4 ounces cooked chicken, shredded

1 onion, finely chopped

1 red bell pepper, chopped

1 green bell pepper, chopped

1½ cups frozen corn, thawed

1 garlic clove, minced

Juice of 1 lime

½ teaspoon chili powder

Pinch sea salt

¼ cup fresh cilantro, chopped

Quesadillas are easy and popular with kids and adults alike. Stop by the grocery store and pick up a precooked rotisserie chicken (or use leftover chicken) to make this super fast. The cooked salsa is a perfect complement and adds lots of bright color.

1. Preheat the oven to 450°F.
2. Using 2 tablespoons of the olive oil, brush one side of each tortilla with the oil. Place 4 of the tortillas oiled side down on a rimmed baking sheet.
3. Sprinkle with the cheese and top with the chicken. Top each with the remaining tortillas, oiled side up.
4. Bake for about 10 minutes, until the cheese is melted and the tortillas toasty. Cut into wedges to serve.
5. While the tortillas cook, in a large, nonstick skillet, heat the remaining 2 tablespoons of olive oil on medium high until it shimmers.
6. Add the onion, bell peppers, and corn, and cook, stirring occasionally, for about 5 minutes, until soft. Add the garlic and cook, stirring constantly, for 30 seconds. Remove a toddler portion and spoon over your toddler's quesadilla.
7. Add the lime juice, chili powder, and salt. Cook, stirring, for 1 minute more.
8. Stir in the cilantro off the heat. You can sprinkle a little cilantro on the toddler portion if desired. Spoon the salsa over the quesadillas to serve.

SUBSTITUTION TIP: Not everyone likes the flavor of cilantro and some people find it soapy tasting, which is actually a genetic trait. You can replace the cilantro with an equal amount of chopped fresh parsley or omit it altogether.

Peanut Butter Noodles with Chicken

`DF`

SERVES 4

PREP TIME: 10 MINUTES
COOK TIME: 10 MINUTES

1 (8-ounce) package buckwheat noodles

½ cup unsalted vegetable broth

1 tablespoon fresh ginger, grated

2 scallions, both white and green parts, finely chopped

1 garlic clove, peeled

2 tablespoons tamari or reduced-sodium soy sauce

Juice of 1 lime

¼ cup peanut butter

1 tablespoon honey (optional)

8 ounces cooked chicken meat, shredded or chopped

This is another really quick meal that you can serve hot or cold. You can use leftover chicken or buy a precooked rotisserie chicken, which makes it even faster since all you need to cook is the noodles. Even without the added meat, the peanut butter gives the noodles a protein-infusion. Add steamed veggies for an even more nutritious meal.

1. Cook the noodles according to the package directions, drain, and set aside.
2. In a blender or food processor, combine the vegetable broth, ginger, scallions, garlic, tamari, lime juice, peanut butter, and honey (if using). Process until smooth. Transfer to a small saucepan.
3. Heat on medium high, stirring constantly, until warm.
4. In a large bowl, toss with the chicken and hot noodles.

SUBSTITUTION TIP: If you don't have buckwheat noodles on hand and everyone in your family tolerates gluten, you can instead use whole-wheat spaghetti noodles. If gluten is problematic, be sure to select a brand of buckwheat noodles that are gluten-free, as many types contain both buckwheat and wheat. For peanut allergies, substitute almond butter, sun butter, or cashew butter for the peanut butter. To make it vegan, omit the honey.

Chicken Chow Mein

DF NF

SERVES 4

PREP TIME: 10 MINUTES
COOK TIME: 10 MINUTES

1 (8-ounce) package rice noodles or soba noodles

2 tablespoons coconut oil

8 ounces boneless, skinless chicken breasts or thighs, cut into ½-inch pieces

1 onion, finely chopped

1 teaspoon fresh ginger, grated

1 cup Napa cabbage or green cabbage, shredded

2 carrots, peeled and grated

3 scallions, finely chopped

3 garlic cloves, minced

2 tablespoons tamari

2 teaspoons cornstarch

1 teaspoon sesame oil

1 teaspoon honey

¼ cup unsalted vegetable broth

This quick stir-fry uses rice noodles or soba noodles for a fun and easy one-dish meal. If gluten isn't an issue and you can't find rice or gluten-free soba noodles, you can use whole-wheat spaghetti or angel hair instead.

1. Cook the noodles according to the package directions, drain, and set aside.

2. In a large pot or nonstick skillet, heat the coconut oil on medium high until it shimmers.

3. Add the chicken and cook for about 5 minutes, stirring occasionally, until cooked through. Using a slotted spoon, remove the chicken from the oil and set aside.

4. Add the onion and ginger to the oil and cook for about 4 minutes, stirring occasionally, until the onion softens.

5. Add the cabbage, carrots, and scallions. Cook for 3 minutes, stirring occasionally. Add the garlic and cook, stirring constantly, for 30 seconds.

6. In a small bowl, whisk together the tamari, cornstarch, sesame oil, honey, and vegetable broth. Add to a pot with the cooked noodles. Bring to a simmer. Serve hot.

SUBSTITUTION TIP: To make this vegan, replace the chicken with 8 ounces of chopped tofu.

Slow Cooker BBQ Pulled Chicken

DF GF **NF**

SERVES 4 TO 6

PREP TIME: 10 MINUTES
COOK TIME: 8 HOURS

1½ pounds of boneless, skinless chicken thighs

1 onion, sliced

1 (14-ounce) can tomato sauce

¼ cup pure maple syrup

¼ cup apple cider vinegar

1 teaspoon onion powder

1 teaspoon garlic powder

1 teaspoon chili powder (optional)

1 teaspoon smoked paprika

½ teaspoon liquid smoke

½ teaspoon sea salt

Most commercial barbecue sauces are pretty high in sugar, but in this version you make your own quickly. No need to cook it because in the slow cooker it simmers and blends the flavors well. Serve on buns or in a bowl topped with shredded cabbage for a full meal. If you are concerned about the spice level for your toddler, omit or reduce the chili powder.

1. In the slow cooker, combine the chicken and onion.
2. In a small bowl, whisk together the tomato sauce, maple syrup, vinegar, onion powder, garlic powder, chili powder (if using), smoked paprika, liquid smoke, and sea salt.
3. Pour over the chicken and onions, stirring to mix.
4. Cover and cook on low for 8 hours.
5. Shred the chicken with a fork and return it to the sauce.

COOKING TIP: Add texture by making a quick slaw to go on your pulled chicken sandwiches or in a pulled chicken bowl. In a blender, combine ½ avocado, 2 tablespoons apple cider vinegar, 1 minced garlic clove, and ¼ teaspoon sea salt and blend well. Toss with 2 cups shredded cabbage or premade coleslaw mix.

INGREDIENT TIP: Liquid smoke can be found in the spice aisle of most supermarkets. It is typically smoke that is condensed and added to a liquid medium, usually water. It is a common ingredient in barbecue sauce recipes as it adds the smoky element that gives the barbecue sauce its distinctive flavor. By making your own sauce in this recipe, you reduce the amount of added sugar found in commercially prepared sauces.

Almond-Crusted Chicken Fingers

DF GF

SERVES 4

PREP TIME: 10 MINUTES
COOK TIME: 25 MINUTES

1½ cups almond flour

1 teaspoon dried thyme

½ teaspoon sea salt

¼ teaspoon freshly
ground black pepper

2 large eggs, beaten

1 teaspoon
Dijon mustard

1½ pounds boneless,
skinless chicken
breast tenders

This makes a great meal when cooked fresh, but you can also make a double or triple batch, cook them, freeze them, and reheat them in the oven from frozen. They will freeze well for up to 6 months. Serve with a steamed veggie or as part of a sandwich or slider for a quick lunch or dinner. Cut them into small pieces for toddlers.

1. Preheat the oven to 425°F.
2. In a large bowl, whisk together the almond flour, thyme, salt, and pepper.
3. In a small bowl, whisk together the eggs and mustard.
4. Dip the tenders in the egg mixture and then roll in the almond flour mixture. Place the chicken tenders in a single layer on a rimmed baking sheet.
5. Bake for about 25 minutes, flipping once, until the chicken is golden and cooked.

COOKING TIP: You can reheat these chicken fingers from frozen in a 425°F oven for 20 to 25 minutes. Make a dipping sauce by mixing together ¼ cup plain Greek yogurt, 1 tablespoon Dijon or yellow mustard, and 1 tablespoon honey.

SUBSTITUTION TIP: If nuts are an issue, you can replace the almond flour with an equal amount of bread crumbs.

Roast Chicken and Root Vegetables

DF GF **NF**

SERVES 4 TO 6

PREP TIME: 10 MINUTES
COOK TIME: 1 HOUR
30 MINUTES

1 (5- to 6-pound)
whole chicken

½ teaspoon sea salt

¼ teaspoon freshly
ground black pepper

1 yellow onion, halved

1 fresh thyme bunch

2 garlic cloves, peeled

1 lemon, halved

1 red onion,
roughly chopped

3 carrots, peeled and
roughly chopped

1 fennel bulb, cored and
roughly chopped

1 pound baby red
potatoes or fingerling
potatoes, quartered

2 tablespoons extra-
virgin olive oil

1 teaspoon dried thyme

This is the traditional American supper, and given the long cooking time for the chicken, it's a great weekend meal. Leftover chicken can be shredded and frozen for up to 6 months for use in other recipes.

1. Preheat the oven to 425°F.
2. Remove the giblets from the center of the chicken and rinse and pat the chicken dry. Season with the salt and pepper.
3. In the chicken's cavity, stuff the yellow onion, fresh thyme, garlic, and lemon. Tuck the wing tips under the chicken.
4. In a large bowl, toss the red onion, carrots, fennel, and red potatoes with the olive oil and thyme. Transfer to a roasting pan. Place the chicken on a rack over the vegetables.
5. Bake for about 1 hour and 30 minutes, until the thigh registers 165°F on an instant read thermometer and juices run clear. Allow the chicken to rest for 20 minutes before carving.

COOKING TIP: You can speed up cooking time by using chicken pieces in place of the whole chicken. Drumsticks work well here. Season the drumsticks with salt and pepper (omit the herbs and veggies you would stuff in the chicken's cavity) and arrange them on the root veggies in the roasting pan. Cook for about 25 minutes or until the juices run clear and internal temperature is 165°F.

Ground Turkey and Veggie Skillet

DF GF **NF**

SERVES 4 TO 6

PREP TIME: 10 MINUTES
COOK TIME: 15 MINUTES

2 tablespoons extra-
virgin olive oil

1 pound ground turkey

1 onion, finely chopped

2 carrots, peeled and
finely chopped

1 broccoli bunch,
separated into
small florets

1 cup green cabbage,
shredded

1 teaspoon dried
rosemary

1 (14-ounce) can crushed
tomatoes

¼ cup unsalted
chicken broth

½ teaspoon sea salt

¼ teaspoon freshly
ground black pepper

Mixing ground meats and veggies in a skillet makes a quick, super conve-
nient, and versatile meal. The meat cooks quickly, and it's easy to change
vegetables and herbs. Serve with Cauliflower Rice (page 144) or steamed
brown rice for a full meal.

1. In a large, nonstick skillet, heat the olive oil on medium high until it
shimmers.

2. Add the turkey and cook for about 5 minutes, crumbling with a spoon,
until it is browned. Using a slotted spoon, remove the turkey from the pan
and set it aside.

3. Add the onion, carrots, and broccoli to the pan and cook for about 5 minutes, stirring occasionally, until the veggies are tender. Add the cabbage and
rosemary and cook until the cabbage softens, 2 to 3 minutes more. Add the
tomatoes with their juices, chicken broth, salt, and pepper. Bring to a simmer and remove from the heat to serve.

COOKING TIP: To make this vegetarian, replace the ground turkey with chopped
tofu and the chicken broth with vegetable broth.

Zucchini Noodles with
Slow Cooker Turkey Meatball Marinara

SERVES 4 TO 6

PREP TIME: 10 MINUTES
COOK TIME: 8 HOURS

1 pound ground turkey

½ cup gluten-free
bread crumbs

1 large egg, beaten

1 carrot, peeled
and grated

½ teaspoon sea salt

2 teaspoons dried Italian
herbs, divided

2 (14-ounce) cans
crushed tomatoes,
1 drained

1 onion, finely chopped

1 teaspoon garlic powder

¼ cup fresh
basil, chopped

2 portions Veggie
Noodles (Zoodles)
(page 145)

Making a meatball marinara in the slow cooker is a great way to have a quick dinner for busy weeknights. You can make the meatballs the night before, refrigerate them overnight, and then pop them in the slow cooker with the marinara sauce in the morning so you're not pressed for time.

1. In a large bowl, mix together the ground turkey, bread crumbs, egg, carrot, sea salt, and 1 teaspoon of Italian herbs. Using a melon baller, form the mixture into balls and arrange in the slow cooker.
2. Add the drained tomatoes and one can with its juices, onion, garlic powder, and remaining 1 teaspoon of Italian herbs.
3. Cover and cook on low for 8 hours.
4. Stir in the basil just before serving.
5. Spoon over the zoodles.

COOKING TIP: If desired, you can add up to two cups of additional chopped, fresh veggies to the marinara sauce when you add the other ingredients. Carrots, zucchini, and yellow squash are all good choices.

Turkey Burger with Avocado Sauce

DF NF

SERVES 4

PREP TIME: 10 MINUTES
COOK TIME: 10 MINUTES

1 pound ground turkey

1 teaspoon fish sauce

2 garlic cloves,
minced, divided

1 teaspoon honey

1 carrot, grated

½ onion, grated

2 tablespoons extra-
virgin olive oil

1 avocado

1 tablespoon
Worcestershire sauce

1 tablespoon tamari

1 tablespoon pure
maple syrup

1 tablespoon fresh
chives, chopped

Grating up veggies in turkey burgers adds flavor and nutrition, and it can help keep the burgers moist. Serve on a whole-grain or gluten-free hamburger bun or by itself as a patty with the sauce spooned over the top.

1. In a large bowl, combine the ground turkey, fish sauce, half of the garlic, the honey, carrot, and onion. Mix and form into 4 patties.

2. In a large, nonstick skillet, heat the olive oil on medium high until it shimmers. Add the patties and cook for about 5 minutes per side, flipping once, until cooked through.

3. In a blender or food processor, combine the avocado, Worcestershire sauce, tamari, maple syrup, chives, and remaining minced garlic clove. Blend until smooth.

4. Serve the sauce with the burgers.

COOKING TIP: You can also make the turkey mixture into melon-ball-size meatballs and bake in a 400°F oven for 20 to 25 minutes and serve the avocado sauce on the side for dipping. For fish allergies, replace the fish sauce with tamari and omit the Worcestershire sauce.

Turkey Chili

SERVES 4 TO 6

PREP TIME: 10 MINUTES
COOK TIME: 25 MINUTES

2 tablespoons extra-virgin olive oil

1½ pounds
ground turkey

1 onion, finely chopped

1 green bell pepper,
finely chopped

2 (14-ounce) cans kidney
or pinto beans, drained

2 (14-ounce) cans
crushed tomatoes,
1 drained

1 teaspoon dried oregano

1 teaspoon garlic powder

1 teaspoon ground cumin

½ teaspoon sea salt

1 tablespoon chili powder

If your toddler doesn't like spice and you do, this is an easy recipe to customize. For a spicier chili, remove your toddler's portion then add up to ¼ teaspoon of cayenne pepper. Allow the chili to simmer with the cayenne for another 5 minutes to allow the flavors to blend. This freezes well so make a double batch for an easy meal later.

1. In a large pot, heat the olive oil on medium high until it shimmers. Add the ground turkey and cook for about 5 minutes, crumbling with a spoon, until browned.

2. Add the onion and bell pepper and cook for about 5 minutes, stirring occasionally, until the vegetables soften.

3. Add the kidney beans, drained tomatoes without juices and the can with its juices, oregano, garlic powder, cumin, and salt. Cook for about 10 minutes, stirring occasionally, until the flavors blend well. Remove a toddler portion and set aside.

4. Add the chili powder and cook for 3 minutes more to allow flavors to blend.

COOKING TIP: Garnish with grated cheese, sour cream, and chopped avocados.

Family Taco Night

NF

SERVES 4 TO 6

PREP TIME: 10 MINUTES
COOK TIME: 15 MINUTES

1 pound ground beef

1 onion, finely chopped

1 teaspoon dried oregano

1 teaspoon ground cumin

½ teaspoon ground coriander

½ teaspoon sea salt

1 teaspoon chili powder

1 package corn or whole-wheat tortillas, heated according to package instructions

2 cups lettuce, shredded

1 cup tomatoes, chopped

1 avocado, diced

1 cup Cheddar cheese, grated

1 cup sour cream or plain Greek yogurt

1 cup salsa

Invite family participation in meal prep by making it taco night. Put out various ingredients and garnishes and allow everyone to make their own taco. For your toddler, you may just want to serve meat, cheese, and finely chopped veggies, or you can wrap the meat and cheese in a tortilla and cut into small slices.

1. In a large nonstick skillet on medium-high heat, cook the ground beef for about 5 minutes, crumbling with a spoon, until it is browned.
2. Add the onion and cook for about 5 minutes, stirring occasionally, until softened.
3. Add the oregano, cumin, coriander, salt, and ¼ cup water. Bring to a simmer and reduce the heat. Cook for about 3 minutes more, until the liquid reduces by half. Remove a toddler portion and set aside.
4. Add the chili powder and cook, stirring, for 2 minutes more.
5. Place the tortillas, beef, lettuce, tomatoes, avocado, cheese, sour cream, and salsa out in separate bowls and allow your family to make their own tacos.

SUBSTITUTION TIP: Use any ground meat you choose here. You can also replace the ground beef with chopped tofu. Cook the onion in 2 tablespoons of olive oil and add the tofu. Cook until it is browned, about 5 minutes. Then add seasonings and water and simmer for 3 to 4 minutes.

Gyro Wraps with Tzatziki and Cucumber–Red Onion Quick Pickles

NF

SERVES 4 TO 6

PREP TIME: 20 MINUTES
COOK TIME: 1 HOUR

1 red onion,
roughly chopped

¼ cup fresh
rosemary leaves

¼ cup fresh
oregano leaves

¼ cup fresh
marjoram leaves

4 garlic cloves, peeled

1 pound ground lamb

½ teaspoon sea salt

1 cup plain Greek whole-
milk yogurt

1 cucumber, peeled
and grated

Juice of 1 lemon

1 cup red wine vinegar

1 teaspoon kosher salt

1 red onion, thinly sliced

1 cucumber, peeled and
thinly sliced

4 to 6 whole-wheat wraps

You'll need a food processor to mix up the gyro meat. It takes about an hour to cook in the oven, but it keeps well so you can make it ahead, slice it, and reheat it for quick weeknight meals. Make the tzatziki and quick pickles just before serving. For your toddler, serve the meat and tzatziki sauce over cooked brown rice, Cauliflower Rice (see page 144), or couscous. Omit the wrap and the pickle for toddlers.

1. Preheat the oven to 400°F.
2. In a food processor, process the onion until finely chopped. Turn it out onto a tea towel and roll it in the towel, wringing out excess moisture over the sink. Wipe out the food processor to remove moisture. Return the onion to the food processor.
3. Add the rosemary, oregano, marjoram, garlic, lamb, and salt. Process until well combined, about 4 minutes. Press into a loaf pan.
4. Cook for about 1 hour, until the internal temperature reaches 165°F. Allow to rest for 10 minutes before slicing thinly.
5. Meanwhile, while the gyro cooks, in a small bowl whisk together the yogurt, cucumber, and lemon juice to make the tzatziki. Set aside.
6. In a small bowl, whisk together the red wine vinegar and salt. Add the sliced onion and sliced cucumber to the vinegar and allow to sit at room temperature until the gyro is ready.
7. To serve, slice the gyro thinly and place on the wraps. Top with the tzatziki and quick pickles.

SUBSTITUTION TIP: You can also use ground beef, turkey, or chicken in place of the ground lamb. Cooking time and temperature remain the same for any ground meat.

Asian Ground Pork Stir-Fry with Rice Noodles

SERVES 4 TO 6

PREP TIME: 15 MINUTES
COOK TIME: 15 MINUTES

1 (8-ounce) package
rice noodles

1 Asian pear, peeled,
cored, and chopped

Juice of 1 orange

2 tablespoons tamari

1 teaspoon sesame oil

1 pound ground pork

8 ounces shiitake
mushrooms, stemmed
and thinly sliced

1 scallion bunch, both
white and green parts,
thinly sliced on the bias

4 carrots, peeled
and grated

1 teaspoon fresh
ginger, grated

2 garlic cloves, minced

1 teaspoon Sriracha or
gochujang (optional)

Ground meat stir-fries with veggies quickly. You can serve it with the rice noodles as suggested here, or spoon it over Cauliflower Rice (page 144) or cooked brown rice. Feel free to change the veggies to what is fresh and in season. For your toddler, remove their portion before you stir in the gochujang or Sriracha unless your toddler likes spice.

1. Cook the rice noodles according to the package directions, drain, and set aside.
2. In a blender or food processor, combine the pear, orange juice, tamari, and sesame oil. Blend until smooth.
3. In a large, nonstick skillet, cook the ground pork for about 5 minutes, crumbling with a spoon, until browned.
4. Add the shiitake, scallion, carrots, and ginger. Cook for about 5 minutes more, stirring occasionally, until the veggies soften.
5. Add the garlic and cook, stirring constantly, for 30 seconds.
6. Add the sauce from the food processor. Bring to a simmer and cook for 3 minutes. Separate a toddler's portion and set aside.
7. Stir in the Sriracha (if using). Cook, stirring, for 2 minutes more.
8. Serve over the hot noodles.

SUBSTITUTION TIP: You can also use Veggie Noodles (Zoodles) (page 145) in place of the rice noodles and any other ground meat in place of the pork.

Pork Fried Rice

SERVES 4 TO 6

PREP TIME: 15 MINUTES
COOK TIME: 15 MINUTES

½ pound ground pork

6 scallions, both white
and green parts, thinly
sliced on the bias

1 carrot, peeled
and chopped

1 teaspoon fresh
ginger, grated

1 cup fresh or
frozen peas

1 garlic clove, minced

2 large eggs, beaten

3 cups cooked brown rice

2 tablespoons tamari

Fried rice makes a great hearty meal, or in smaller portions, it's an excellent side dish. Buy your rice precooked so the recipe is quick and easy. Alternatively, you can make it with Cauliflower Rice (page 144).

1. In a large, nonstick skillet or wok, cook the ground pork for about 5 minutes, crumbling with a spoon, until it is browned.
2. Add the scallions, carrot, ginger, and peas. Cook for about 4 minutes, stirring occasionally, until the vegetables are tender.
3. Add the garlic and cook, stirring constantly, for 30 seconds.
4. Add the eggs and cook for about 2 minutes more, stirring, until set.
5. Stir in the rice and tamari until mixed well. Serve.

SUBSTITUTION TIP: To make this vegetarian, replace the ground pork with 8 ounces of chopped tofu and cook it with the vegetables in 2 tablespoons of olive oil for about 5 minutes.

Cheeseburger Sliders with Slow Cooker Caramelized Onions

NF

SERVES 4

PREP TIME: 15 MINUTES
COOK TIME: 8 HOURS

2 yellow onions, very
thinly sliced

2 tablespoons extra-
virgin olive oil

½ teaspoon dried thyme

½ teaspoon sea salt

1 pound ground beef

½ cup Swiss
cheese, grated

½ cup mayonnaise

1 tablespoon soy sauce
or tamari

1 tablespoon
brown sugar

1 garlic clove,
finely minced

1 tablespoon fresh
thyme, chopped

8 slider buns, toasted

Rich, sweet caramelized onions add tremendous flavor to these cheese-burger sliders. Fortunately, you can make them in the slow cooker, and they'll keep in your fridge for 5 days or the freezer for up to 6 months. I recommend making a big batch and thawing them as you need. They are also delicious in omelets, with scrambled eggs, or to make virtually any sandwich or burger more flavorful.

1. In a slow cooker, toss the onions with the olive oil, thyme, and salt. Cover and cook on low for 8 hours. Uncover and cook on high for another 30 minutes.

2. Form 8 patties from the ground beef. Heat a nonstick skillet on medium high. Cook the patties for about 4 minutes per side, flipping once, until cooked through.

3. Sprinkle the cheese over the patties. Turn off the heat and cover, allowing the cheese to melt as the pan cools.

4. In a small bowl, whisk together the mayonnaise, soy sauce, brown sugar, garlic, and thyme. Spread on the buns. Top the buns with a patty and the caramelized onions.

SUBSTITUTION TIP: For gluten-free, use gluten-free slider buns or large pieces of butter lettuce to make a lettuce wrap. You can also make the sliders into meatballs (fold the grated cheese and caramelized onions into the ground beef), bake them for 1 hour in a 350°F oven, and serve them with the mayonnaise mixture as a dipping sauce.

Baked Ziti with Meat Sauce

NF

SERVES 6 TO 8

PREP TIME: 15 MINUTES
COOK TIME: 45 MINUTES

8 ounces whole-wheat rotini pasta

1 pound ground beef

1 onion, finely chopped

1 (14-ounce) can crushed tomatoes, drained

1 (14-ounce) can tomato sauce

1 tablespoon dried Italian herbs

1 teaspoon garlic powder

½ teaspoon sea salt

1 cup Monterey Jack cheese, grated

This freezes well, and it makes a pretty good-sized batch, so it's an excellent make-ahead meal. Make it on the weekend and refrigerate it for up to 5 days or freeze it in single servings for up to 6 months.

1. Preheat the oven to 350°F.
2. Cook the rotini according to the package directions, drain, and set aside.
3. In a large, nonstick skillet, cook the ground beef on medium high for about 5 minutes, crumbling with a spoon, until browned.
4. Add the onion and cook for about 3 minutes more, until softened.
5. Add the crushed tomatoes, tomato sauce, Italian herbs, garlic powder, and salt. Bring to a simmer and cook for 5 minutes, stirring occasionally.
6. Transfer the cooked pasta to a 9-by-13-inch baking pan. Pour the sauce over the top evenly.
7. Top with the cheese. Bake for 45 minutes, until the cheese is bubbly.

SUBSTITUTION TIP: You can use gluten-free pasta in place of the whole-wheat rotini if desired.

Slow Cooker Barley Beef Stew

DF NF

SERVES 6 TO 8

PREP TIME: 15 MINUTES
COOK TIME: 10 HOURS

3 pounds beef stew meat,
cut into 1-inch pieces

1 onion, chopped

2 carrots, peeled
and chopped

8 ounces mushrooms,
quartered

1 cup pearl barley

5 cups unsalted chicken
or beef broth

1 teaspoon garlic powder

1 teaspoon dried
rosemary

1 teaspoon dried thyme

1 teaspoon
Dijon mustard

½ teaspoon sea salt

⅛ teaspoon freshly
ground black pepper

1 cup frozen or
fresh peas

2 tablespoons cornstarch

1 tablespoon fresh
parsley, chopped

Stew meat does well in a slow cooker because it requires low, slow cooking to break down the collagen and render it tender. If your store doesn't have stew meat, you can also use chuck roast that you've cut into cubes. Remember barley isn't gluten-free, so if gluten is an issue, you'll want to omit the barley and stir in some other cooked grain before serving. For your toddler, you'll likely want to cut the meat into smaller pieces

1. In a slow cooker, combine the beef, onion, carrots, mushrooms, pearl barley, chicken broth, garlic powder, rosemary, thyme, mustard, salt, and pepper. Cover and cook on low for 8 to 10 hours.
2. When cooking is complete, add the peas. In a small bowl, whisk together the cornstarch and 2 tablespoons water. Stir into the stew. Turn the slow cooker to high and cook, uncovered, stirring occasionally, for about 30 minutes more, until the stew thickens.
3. Stir in the parsley before serving.

SUBSTITUTION TIP: You can enjoy this as more of a soupy stew and save time by omitting the cornstarch and water. Instead, after 8 to 10 hours, stir in the peas, cover, and cook for about 10 minutes more to allow the peas to cook through.

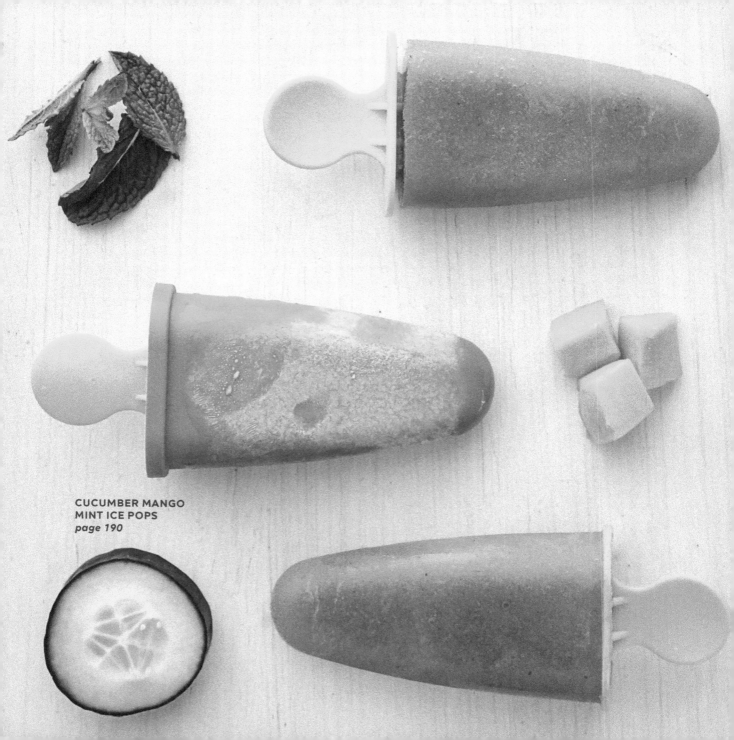

CUCUMBER MANGO
MINT ICE POPS
page 190

10
SWEET TREATS

Sweets are best used as a sometimes treat—unless they are 100 percent fruit. Using too much sugar replaces nutrient-dense foods with empty calorie foods, and serving overly sweet foods can lead to a lifetime of sweets cravings. Most days of the week, offer fruit as treats. However, once or twice a week a low-sugar sweet, especially those included here, can be part of a nutritious eating pattern for your toddler.

Cucumber Mango Mint Ice Pops

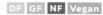

SERVES 4

PREP TIME: 10 MINUTES,
PLUS ABOUT 6 HOURS
FREEZING TIME

1 cucumber, peeled
and chopped

1 mango, peeled
and cubed

1 tablespoon fresh
mint, chopped

1 cup apple juice or
white grape juice

I especially love ice pops for toddlers because they are refreshing, easy to eat, and you can incorporate so many healthy ingredients in them and still have them taste great. They're also a great snack for when your little one has molars popping in that are bothering her.

1. In a blender or food processor, combine the cucumber, mango, mint, and juice. Blend until smooth.
2. Pour into a four-serving ice pop mold and freeze for about 6 hours, or until frozen.

COOKING TIP: If you don't have an ice pop mold, you can use paper cups. Pour the mixture in the cups and cover them with foil. Then, poke the sticks through the foil into the ice pops. The foil will hold the sticks in place while the ice pops freeze.

Dairy-Free Fudgesicles

SERVES 4

PREP TIME: 5 MINUTES,
PLUS ABOUT 6 HOURS
FREEZING TIME

1 cup canned
coconut milk

½ cup unsweetened
cacao powder

6 tablespoons pure
maple syrup

These creamy treats are the perfect alternative to ice cream. Your toddler will love them, and he can help you make them by measuring ingredients and whisking the mixture until it's blended. These fudgesicles are also naturally sweetened with maple syrup.

1. In a liquid measuring cup, whisk together the coconut milk, cacao powder, and maple syrup until well combined.
2. Pour into a four-serving ice pop mold and freeze for about 6 hours, or until frozen.

VARIATION TIP: You can add 3 tablespoons of nut butter, such as peanut butter. If you do, blend well in a blender or food processor instead of whisking to ensure the nut butter is mixed well.

INGREDIENT TIP: When using canned coconut milk, shake well to ensure it is well blended and always store in the cupboard and not the fridge. Storing it in the fridge can cause the solids to separate from the liquid. If the resulting flavor is too strongly coconut, you can replace with another nondairy milk, such as almond milk.

Avocado Chocolate Mousse

SERVES 2

PREP TIME: 5 MINUTES

1 avocado

2 tablespoons pure
maple syrup

¼ cup unsweetened
cacao powder

2 tablespoons nondairy
milk (see page 76) or
whole milk

½ teaspoon
vanilla extract

Pinch salt

Who knew avocado would work so well in sweet pudding-like recipes? Its creamy consistency makes it the perfect base for a sweet chocolate mousse that's dairy- and cooking-free, and perfectly creamy and smooth.

In a blender or food processor, combine the avocado, maple syrup, cacao powder, milk, vanilla, and salt. Blend until smooth and serve.

INGREDIENT TIP: Choose an avocado that has a slight give when gently pressed with the thumb but not one that is so soft it squishes under your thumb. You can also flick the stem end off and look to make sure the flesh underneath is green instead of brown. If it's brown, it's overripe.

Banana-Pineapple Ice Cream Sundaes

SERVES 4

PREP TIME: 5 MINUTES
COOK TIME: 5 MINUTES

**2 tablespoons
unsalted butter**

1 banana, sliced

**1 cup fresh or canned
and drained pineapple,
finely chopped**

¼ cup pure maple syrup

**½ teaspoon
ground ginger**

Pinch salt

1 pint vanilla ice cream

Make this simple banana-pineapple sauce and store it in the fridge for up to 5 days, reheating it on the stove top or in the microwave before spooning it over ice cream. Julian loves to help me make this fruity sauce and the banana is perfect for little fingers to practice their chopping skills with a butter knife.

1. In a large, nonstick skillet, melt the butter on medium high until it bubbles.

2. Add the banana and pineapple and cook for about 5 minutes, stirring occasionally, until the fruit begins to brown.

3. Add the maple syrup, ginger, and salt. Simmer for 3 minutes. Serve spooned over the ice cream.

SUBSTITUTION TIP: You can also serve this spooned over plain unsweetened yogurt like you would with a fruit parfait. This has less sugar than ice cream.

Yogurt Bark

GF NF V

SERVES 4

PREP TIME: 5 MINUTES,
PLUS 4 HOURS
FREEZING TIME

2 cups plain whole-
milk yogurt

2 tablespoons honey

1 teaspoon
vanilla extract

2 tablespoons
chocolate chips

2 tablespoons chopped
strawberries

2 tablespoons pumpkin
seeds (optional)

I love yogurt bark. This colorful, simple, and fun recipe makes for a great snack, treat, or even breakfast. It's naturally high in protein, low in sugar, and great for kids and adults. Use whole-milk yogurt to ensure the creamiest taste!

1. In a small bowl, mix the yogurt, honey, and vanilla. Pour onto a parchment paper-lined baking sheet.
2. Sprinkle the chocolate chips, strawberries, and/or pumpkin seeds (if using) on top.
3. Freeze for at least 4 hours. Once frozen, break into pieces and transfer to an airtight container and store in the freezer.

SUBSTITUTION TIP: You can play around with all sorts of toppings on these, so just use your imagination to create your favorite bark. Crushed almonds and pistachios are great sprinkled on top, as are dried berries, seeds, and even spices like cinnamon and nutmeg.

Strawberries with Mexican Chocolate Yogurt Dip

SERVES 2

PREP TIME: 5 MINUTES

½ cup plain whole-
milk yogurt

2 tablespoons
unsweetened
cacao powder

1 tablespoon pure
maple syrup

¼ teaspoon ground
cinnamon

Pinch allspice

1 cup sliced strawberries

Mexican hot chocolate has a touch of cinnamon and allspice in it to give it extra flavor. In some cases, it also has a pinch cayenne for heat, which we will omit here. This slightly spicy, sweet dip is packed with the flavors of Mexican hot chocolate and your little one will love it for dipping sliced strawberries or other fruits.

1. In a small bowl, whisk together the yogurt, cacao powder, maple syrup, cinnamon, and allspice.
2. Serve with the strawberries (or another sliced fruit) for dipping.

SUBSTITUTION TIP: You can also use unsweetened carob powder in place of the cacao powder.

Banana Ice Cream with Chocolate Sauce

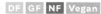

SERVES 4

PREP TIME: 5 MINUTES

2 bananas, sliced
and frozen

¼ cup melted coconut oil

2 tablespoons pure
maple syrup

2 tablespoons
unsweetened
cacao powder

Pinch sea salt

Mix up a quick batch of this banana ice cream, which has only one ingredient: bananas. The ice cream is creamy and delicious, and when topped with a little chocolate sauce, it's the perfect nutritious sweet bite for your toddler.

1. In a blender or food processor, blend the bananas until smooth.
2. In a small bowl, whisk together the coconut oil, maple syrup, cacao powder, and salt.
3. Spoon the chocolate sauce over the banana ice cream and serve.

INGREDIENT TIP: Store the chocolate sauce at room temperature. If it hardens, reheat in a saucepan over medium-low heat, stirring constantly.

Easy Peanut Butter Cookies

 DF GF V

MAKES 24 COOKIES

PREP TIME: 5 MINUTES
COOK TIME: 15 MINUTES

1 cup peanut butter

¼ cup coconut sugar

1 egg, beaten

1 teaspoon baking soda

These cookies have only four ingredients, and they are gluten-free. While the recipe calls for coconut sugar, which you can find at the health food store or online, you can also use brown or white sugar in its place, if desired. It needs to be a granulated sugar (as opposed to honey or maple syrup) to get the texture right.

1. Preheat the oven to 350°F. Line a baking sheet with parchment paper.
2. In a small bowl or mixer, mix the peanut butter, coconut sugar, egg, and baking soda.
3. Drop in 1-teaspoon balls onto the prepared baking sheet. Flatten slightly with a fork, making a cross-hatch pattern with the tines.
4. Bake for about 10 minutes, until browned.

INGREDIENT TIP: For peanut allergies, almond and cashew butter in the same amount will work well. You can also use crunchy peanut butter to add texture.

Brownies

DF GF V

MAKES 9 BROWNIES

PREP TIME: 15 MINUTES
COOK TIME: 25 MINUTES

¼ cup plus 1 tablespoon coconut oil, plus extra for greasing

¾ cup semisweet chocolate chips or chopped chocolate

¾ cup coconut sugar

2 large eggs, beaten

1½ teaspoons vanilla extract

2 tablespoons unsweetened cacao powder

½ teaspoon baking powder

¾ cup almond flour

Pinch sea salt

This recipe makes fudgy brownies with a nice density. While the recipe calls for coconut sugar, you can also use sugar (in an equal amount) in its place if that's what you choose.

1. Preheat the oven to 350°F. Grease an 8-inch square baking pan with coconut oil.

2. In a small saucepan, heat the chocolate chips, coconut oil, and coconut sugar on medium high, stirring constantly, until melted.

3. Remove from the heat and whisk in the eggs and vanilla.

4. In a small bowl, whisk together the cacao powder, baking powder, almond flour, and salt. Stir into the chocolate mixture until combined.

5. Spread in an even layer in the prepared baking pan. Bake for about 20 minutes, until a toothpick inserted in the center comes out clean. Cool before cutting into squares.

COOKING TIP: You can make releasing the brownies easier by laying two 15-inch-long rectangles of parchment in the baking pan overlapping in a "T" formation so the parchment extends up and over the sides of the pan. No need to grease it before you pour the brownie mix on the parchment in the pan. Then, simply lift out the parchment after the brownies are baked using the extended sides as handles and set them to cool on a wire rack.

Apple Spice Celebration Cake with Maple Cream Cheese Icing

SERVES 10

PREP TIME: 30 MINUTES
COOK TIME: 25 MINUTES

Whether it's a birthday party or some other type of celebration, sometimes only cake will do. In those cases, try this sweet and delicious cake that's lower in processed sugar than many cakes.

FOR THE CAKE

¾ cup coconut oil, melted

½ cup pure maple syrup

¼ cup unsweetened applesauce

2 large eggs, beaten

1 teaspoon vanilla extract

1½ cups cake flour

¼ cup coconut sugar

½ teaspoon baking powder

½ teaspoon baking soda

Pinch sea salt

1 teaspoon ground ginger

1 teaspoon ground cinnamon

½ teaspoon ground cloves

2 apples, peeled, cored, and finely chopped

FOR THE FROSTING

6 ounces cream cheese, softened

3 tablespoons unsalted butter, softened

¼ cup pure maple syrup

¼ teaspoon vanilla extract

TO MAKE THE CAKE

1. Preheat the oven to 325°F. Grease and flour two (8-inch) round layer cake pans.
2. In a large bowl, beat together the coconut oil, maple syrup, applesauce, eggs, and vanilla.
3. In a medium bowl, sift together the cake flour, coconut sugar, baking powder, baking soda, salt, ginger, cinnamon, and cloves.
4. Add the dry ingredients to the wet and mix until just combined. Fold in the apples.
5. Spread evenly in the two prepared cake pans. Bake for about 20 minutes, until a toothpick inserted in the cake comes out clean. Cool on a wire rack.
6. When the cakes have cooled, turn out from the pans and rest on the wire rack until cool before frosting.

TO MAKE THE FROSTING

In a medium bowl, combine the cream cheese, butter, maple syrup, and vanilla. Beat until smooth.

TO ASSEMBLE THE CAKE

1. Set one of the cake rounds on a cake plate and trim the top with a serrated knife to make it even. Using an offset spatula, ice around the sides and the top of the round.
2. Place the other cake round on top. Ice the sides and top.

COOKING TIP: If you like, you can use unsweetened apple butter (commercially prepared or homemade) or an apple purée as the filling between layers. Spread about ½ cup on the bottom layer in place of icing, icing only around the sides of the layer. Then, top with the second layer, and ice the top and sides to hide the filling.

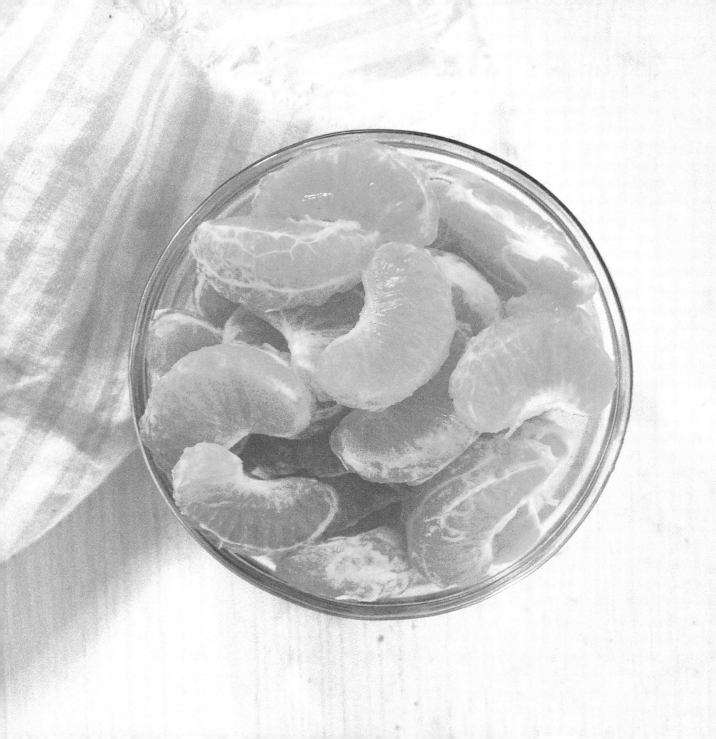

The Dirty Dozen and the Clean Fifteen™

The Environmental Working Group (EWG) is a nonprofit, nonpartisan organization dedicated to protecting human health and the environment. Its mission is to empower people to live healthier lives in a healthier environment. This organization publishes an annual list of the twelve kinds of produce, in sequence, that have the highest amount of pesticide residue—the Dirty Dozen—as well as a list of the fifteen kinds of produce that have the least amount of pesticide residue—the Clean Fifteen.

THE DIRTY DOZEN

The 2018 Dirty Dozen includes the following produce. These are considered the most important produce to buy organically:

1. Strawberries
2. Spinach
3. Nectarines
4. Apples
5. Grapes
6. Peaches
7. Cherries
8. Pears
9. Tomatoes
10. Celery
11. Potatoes
12. Sweet bell peppers
+ Hot peppers*

*The Dirty Dozen list contains one additional item—hot peppers—because they tend to contain trace levels of highly hazardous pesticides.

THE CLEAN FIFTEEN

The least critical to buy organically are the Clean Fifteen list. The following are on the 2018 list:

1. Avocados
2. Sweet Corn
3. Pineapples
4. Cabbages
5. Onions
6. Sweet peas frozen
7. Papayas
8. Asparagus
9. Mangoes
10. Eggplants
11. Honeydew melons
12. Kiwis
13. Cantaloupes
14. Cauliflower
15. Broccoli

Measurement Conversions

VOLUME EQUIVALENTS (LIQUID)

US STANDARD	US STANDARD (ounces)	METRIC (approximate)
2 tablespoons	1 fl. oz.	30 mL
¼ cup	2 fl. oz.	60 mL
½ cup	4 fl. oz.	120 mL
1 cup	8 fl. oz.	240 mL
1½ cups	12 fl. oz.	355 mL
2 cups or 1 pint	16 fl. oz.	475 mL
4 cups or 1 quart	32 fl. oz.	1 L
1 gallon	128 fl. oz.	4 L

OVEN TEMPERATURES

FAHRENHEIT (F)	CELSIUS (C) (approximate)
250°F	120°C
300°F	150°C
325°F	165°C
350°F	180°C
375°F	190°C
400°F	200°C
425°F	220°C
450°F	230°C

VOLUME EQUIVALENTS (DRY)

US STANDARD	METRIC (approximate)	US STANDARD	METRIC (approximate)
⅛ teaspoon	0.5 mL	½ cup	118 mL
¼ teaspoon	1 mL	⅔ cup	156 mL
½ teaspoon	2 mL	¾ cup	177 mL
¾ teaspoon	4 mL	1 cup	235 mL
1 teaspoon	5 mL	2 cups or 1 pint	475 mL
1 tablespoon	15 mL	3 cups	700 mL
¼ cup	59 mL	4 cups or 1 quart	1 L
⅓ cup	79 mL		

WEIGHT EQUIVALENTS

US STANDARD	METRIC (approximate)
½ ounce	15 g
1 ounce	30 g
2 ounces	60 g
4 ounces	115 g
8 ounces	225 g
12 ounces	340 g
16 ounces or 1 pound	455 g

References

Afify, A.E.-M.M.R., H.S. El-Beltagi, S.M. Abd El-Salam, and A.A. Omran. "Bioavailability of Iron, Zinc, Phytate and Phytase Activity During Soaking and Germination of White Sorghum Varieties." *PLoS ONE* 6, no. 10 (2011): e25512. doi:10.1371/journal.pone.0025512.

Barański M., D. Średnicka-Tober, N. Volakakis, C. Seal, R. Sanderson, G.B. Stewart, C. Benbrook, et al. "Higher Antioxidant and Lower Cadmium Concentrations and Lower Incidence of Pesticide Residues in Organically Grown Crops: A Systematic Literature Review and Meta-Analyses." *The British Journal of Nutrition* 112, no. 5 (September 2014): 794–811. doi:10.1017/S0007114514001366.

Greer, F.R. "Issues in Establishing Vitamin D Recommendations for Infants and Children." *American Journal of Clinical Nutrition* 80, 6 suppl. (December 2004): 1759S–1762S. www.ncbi.nlm.nih.gov/pubmed/15585801.

Greer, F.R. and S. Marshall. "Bone Mineral Content, Serum Vitamin D Metabolite Concentrations, and Ultraviolet B Light Exposure in Infants Fed Human Milk With and Without Vitamin D2 Supplements." *The Journal of Pediatrics* 114, no. 2 (1989): 204–212. www.ncbi.nlm.nih.gov/pubmed/2783734.

Kim, M.H. and H. Kim. "The Roles of Glutamine in the Intestine and Its Implication in Intestinal Diseases." *International Journal of Molecular Sciences* 18, no. 5 (May 2017): 1051. doi:10.3390/ijms18051051.

Lönnerdal, Bo. "Calcium and Iron Absorption —Mechanisms and Public Health Relevance." *International Journal for Vitamin and Nutrition Research* 80, no. 45 (2010): 293–299. doi:10.1024/0300-9831/a000036.

Rao, R. and G. Samak. "Role of Glutamine in Protection of Intestinal Epithelial Tight Junctions." *Journal of Epithelial Biology & Pharmacology* 5, suppl. 1-M7 (2012): 47–54. doi:10.2174/1875044301205010047.

Schettle, Lidia, PA-C and Peter A. Lio, MD. "Probiotics: The Search For Bacterial Balance." *The National Eczema Institute.* https://nationaleczema.org/search-bacterial-balance/.

Średnicka-Tober, D., M. Barański, C.J. Seal, R. Sanderson, C. Benbrook, H. Steinshamn, J. Gromadzka-Ostrowska, E. Rembiałkowska, K. Skwarło-Sońta, M. Eyre et al. "Higher PUFA and n-3 PUFA, Conjugated Linoleic Acid, α-tocopherol and Iron, but Lower Iodine and Selenium Concentrations in Organic Milk: A Systematic Literature Review and Meta-and Redundancy Analyses." *British Journal of Nutrition* 115, no. 6 (March 2016): 1043–1060. doi:10.1017/S0007114516000349.

Young, Genevieve S., Julie A. Conquer, and René Thomas. "Effect of Randomized Supplementation with High Dose Olive, Flax or Fish Oil on Serum Phospholipid Fatty Acid Levels in Adults with Attention Deficit Hyperactivity Disorder." *Reproduction, Nutrition, Development* 45, no. 5 (2005): 549–558. doi:10.1051/rnd:2005045.

Index of Recipes by Dietary Label

Index

Acknowledgments

To my son, Julian, you are the inspiration for this book. Your absolute love of life, pure joy, fierce curiosity, but most importantly your beyond-your-years empathy, inspire me every day. To our newest addition, Remi, I love you to pieces and cannot wait to begin our food adventures together. To my husband, without whom none of this would be possible. You taught me to love food and are truly my partner in the kitchen. Your passion and dedication to our children, their health, and palates is remarkable. I am lucky to have you. To my parents, who set a good foundation of healthy eating early and who remind me every day how picky an eater I was. You have always been my most trusted advisors!

To my in-laws, Terry and Linda, the way you care for Julian and Remi is remarkable, they are better having you in their lives.

To Pegah Pjajli, who was a constant support and advisor for this book and my go-to for all things pediatric nutrition. To Sydney Greene, thank you for all your help and for keeping me sane and organized through this whole process. To Beth Lipton, you are incredible and I am so lucky to have you as part of my team. To Eliza Whetzel, thanks for always being my sounding board, you have been a huge asset.

Thank you to my entire team at Callisto Media. It truly has been a collaborative effort. To Elizabeth Castoria, my wonderful editor Salwa Jabado, and to my chef collaborator, Karen Frazier, thanks for helping me bring my vision to life.

About the Author

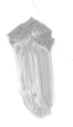

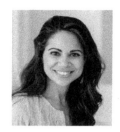

STEPHANIE MIDDLEBERG, MS, RD, CDN, is one of New York City's most sought-after health experts and the bestselling author of *The Big Book of Organic Baby Food*. The founder and owner of Middleberg Nutrition, she and her team of registered dietitians offer nutritional counseling and cooking classes to individuals and families as well as consulting, advising, and planning services to food companies. When she isn't working with her clients or media outlets, Stephanie enjoys eating and playing with her young children, Julian and Remi, jogging with her husband, Andrew, and concocting recipes in the Middleberg Nutrition Test Kitchen. Follow or connect with Stephanie online: ℮ MiddlebergNutrition.com, ⊙ @SMiddleberg_RD, 🐦 @SMiddleberg_RD, and 🅵 facebook.com/MiddlebergNutrition.

Discover More Family Favorites for Babies and Toddlers

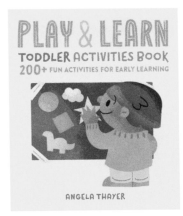

Play & Learn Toddler Activities Book
200+ Fun Activities for Early Learning
Angela Thayer

 ROCKRIDGE PRESS

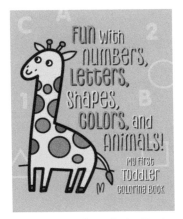

My First Toddler Coloring Book
Fun with Numbers, Letters,
Shapes, Colors, and Animals
Tanya Emelyanova

 ROCKRIDGE PRESS

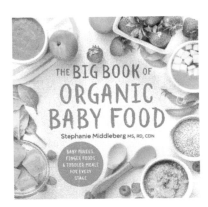

The Big Book of Organic Baby Food
Baby Purées, Finger Foods,
and Toddler Meals For Every Stage
Stephanie Middleberg, MS, RD, CDN

 SONOMA PRESS

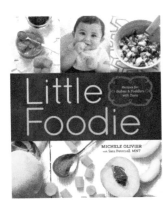

Little Foodie
Baby Food Recipes for Babies
and Toddlers with Taste
Michele Olivier with Sara Peternell

 SONOMA PRESS

CPSIA information can be obtained
at www.ICGtesting.com
Printed in the USA
BVHW05s1418240718
522462BV00001B/1/P